THE
EMERGENCY BOOK

BRADLEY SMITH AND GUS STEVENS

ALLEN LANE

Penguin Handbooks

The Emergency Book

Bradley Smith has also written
The USA: A History in Art, *The Life of the Elephant*,
The Horse in the West and
The New Photography.
He is well known as a photographer for such
magazines as *Life* and *Time*.

Gus Stevens is a feature writer and
columnist for the *San Diego Union Tribune*,
and has also written articles for popular
magazines such as *American Home* and
Town and Country.

ALLEN LANE
Penguin Books Ltd
536 King's Road
London SW10 0UH

First published in the United States by Simon & Schuster 1978
This revised and adapted edition published in Penguin Books 1982
Published by Allen Lane 1982

Copyright © Gemini Smith Inc., 1978, 1982

All rights reserved. No part of this publication
may be reproduced, stored in a retrieval system, or transmitted
in any form or by any means, electronic,
mechanical, photocopying, recording or otherwise, without
the prior permission of the copyright owner.

ISBN 0 7139 1531 5

Set in Ehrhardt and Univers
Printed in Great Britain

This book is dedicated to all those
men and women willing to take the time
and to make the effort to save a life.

Contents

Acknowledgements

Both models used in this book are experienced in the field of emergency medicine: David Chessmore, paramedic, and Cathy Box, nurse, both of Emergency Services, Bay General Community Hospital, Chula Vista, California. Our thanks to both of them and to Melvin A. Ochs, MD, Chairman of Emergency Services, who acted as consultant to the authors.

Foreword

You can save a life. If this opportunity comes to you it can be an experience so rewarding that it can sustain you for the rest of your own life. You will have helped to give the ultimate gift.

Let me tell you what I mean. Not long ago a colleague of mine who is very experienced in saving lives had a heart attack. He suffered a cardiac arrest. His own life hung in the balance. But he was lucky. He was among lay persons – people without formal medical training – who had some knowledge of emergency procedures. They gave my stricken friend mouth-to-mouth respiration and they applied external cardiac compression until professional medical personnel arrived to take charge.

My friend credits these laymen with saving his life. He later said to me, 'To have your life saved is to receive the ultimate gift – and to save a life yourself is the ultimate high. Believe me, I know this and now my laymen friends know it.'

As a doctor I know very well the thrill and feeling of accomplishment these people felt when they realized that, because of what they knew, because of their courage and because of their action they saved a life – the life of a man who recovered and was able to continue his own career in helping others. A vital prerequisite here is knowledge. Without it they wouldn't have been able to act effectively, no matter how much courage and will for action they demonstrated.

In my work in emergency medicine I see a daily procession of misfortune and tragedy, at all hours, day and night. The scene is even more tragic when the family or friends of the victim come to realize that if they had known what to do they might have saved a loved one. To stand by wringing your hands while a life ebbs away is the most helpless and intimidating feeling in the world. I've seen it. I know.

Thankfully, there is another side to the coin. I am delighted when someone has taken the time to learn the basics of emergency medical procedure and has the courage and confidence to ease suffering, minimize injury and, perhaps, even to save the life of an emergency victim. Believe me, I never hesitate to lavish praise on these people. They've earned it.

All of us are Good Samaritans in one way or another, willing to help a friend or a stranger in distress. But the person who takes enough interest in himself, his family and his brother to learn how to save a life – well, these people are the quality people. They're not afraid of life, living their own to the fullest and making it possible for others to do the same.

I have always been fascinated by the number of books available on the subject of helping people to help themselves. So many titles! Diet, meditation, giving up smoking, giving up alcohol, exercising, mental health, getting along with your friends, your mate or your boss – all for your own benefit. Almost none of this material is devoted to the idea of helping others, not even our own families and friends.

In England and Wales more than 100,000 people die each year from heart attacks and more than 17,000 from accidents. We must assume that most of these attacks and accidents happen when there is no trained medical person close by to give instant treatment. How many could be saved if someone with basic medical knowledge were on the scene? Nobody knows exactly, but we do know that a high percentage of these victims would have had at least a chance to survive.

If you have picked up this book and read these early remarks, it means you must have some interest in this subject. Believe me, much of the basic, vital information you can get from this book about the human body and the way it functions will intrigue you – and it will be useful to you in many ways and at many times in your life. The text has been written clearly and with as much basic simplicity as the subject will allow.

I defy anyone to read the chapter about how a baby is born and not be fascinated by the story of how human life begins. Or the dramatic chapter about choking. It shows how fragile our lives really are, how quickly they can end if knowledgeable assistance is not close at hand.

I invite you to invest a little of your time for study and practice so that you will understand a few facts of life – and death – that could help your child, your wife or husband, your parent, your friend, neighbour or someone you may never have met. You may even help yourself when there's nobody else around.

You may never be called on to use what you learn about emergency first aid procedures. But as long as man lives his life the way he does, you must face the possibility. Let us also understand that these procedures are basic emergency measures which should be used only in situations when there is no professional medical person present, and when there is little likelihood that anybody more competent than you will arrive in time to help. What is important is that you be prepared to help when the need is there.

It's up to you. You can save a life!

Melvin A. Ochs, MD
Chairman,
Emergency Services Department
Bay General Community Hospital
Chula Vista, California

1. You Can Save a Life

You can save a life. That is what this book is all about. In these pages is proof that you do not need to flee an accident in panic. You do not need to stand by helplessly and watch another human being die. You do not need to shrink into the crowd, watching someone else take charge – if there is anyone else. If you are prepared, if you have confidence, if you really care, you can act almost on instinct, instantly, when it counts. You can save a life.

Joe and Alma were driving on the motorway, going to spend the weekend with their daughter. After forty miles Joe felt a sharp pain in his chest, a pain which quickly travelled to his neck and his arms. He was able to slow the car and pull over to the side of the busy motorway, where he stopped safely. But obviously Joe was seriously ill and, Alma saw, helpless. He lapsed into unconsciousness and Alma cried out, hugging him, but there was nothing she could do. His heart was weakening. Leaping from the car, she began in desperation to wave at passing traffic . . .

Sarah was only eight but she was a very good swimmer for her age. Most children who live near water do swim well and a dip in the river seemed safe enough. Sarah waded into the water while her parents were setting up camp on the opposite slope of a hill, just out of sight of the river. Somehow Sarah slipped, floundered and started to gulp a great deal of water. She coughed and spluttered for a minute, unable to get on her feet. Then, quite suddenly, she was unconscious, unseen and quite possibly about to drown . . .

It happened in a fashionable restaurant in a large city. John and his wife were visiting the city and, after two weeks, they were going to drive home the next morning. This was to be a farewell night on the town until their next visit to their son, daughter-in-law and two grandchildren. The foursome was lively, laughing, enjoying memories of years past. Suddenly, John began to cough, but no one thought much about it at first. He had brought a cold with him, and it had been stubbornly refusing to go away. But then John was no longer coughing. He was beginning to turn blue as he clutched at his throat. He lurched out of his seat, and the others, now alarmed, rose with him. But as they reached to help him, he began to slip to the floor. He was quickly losing consciousness . . .

It was a warm afternoon as Fred and Jim drove their van along the narrow lane out in the country. As they passed an isolated house they heard a cry for help. They stopped and listened. The cry – a woman's cry – was repeated. They leaped from the van and rushed to the door. It was unlocked and they cautiously looked inside. On the floor was a pregnant woman, writhing in pain. She saw them and cried, 'Please help me! It's my time! The baby's coming early!'

The names of the people in these stories have been changed to protect their privacy, but each is a true story. In each case someone was threatened by a serious medical emergency. Heart attack, drowning, choking and childbirth unattended. Each was only one of thousands of people stricken by these and other emergencies every year. In every case, as with these people, they were reaching out for help. Would they be among the lucky ones who would find help in time?

It's easy enough to hope for them, to pray for their welfare, to cross your fingers and have faith that a doctor, a lifeguard or somebody else with emergency medical training will come along in time to provide the happy ending. But don't count on it.

The message here is that in our fast-moving, volatile and often dangerous society there simply are not enough professionals handy to take care of these life-and-death emergencies. And these are real emergencies, the kind in which it isn't enough to bundle the victims into a car or ambulance and take them to a hospital. In these cases help is needed right now, in minutes – seconds, even. The sooner the help is given the better the chances that lives can be saved.

So who does that leave? Perhaps you've guessed. It's you. Not your neighbour, not the person in the next car, not the next driver to pass by, not another sunbather, not the fellow eating his dinner at the next table. It's you.

Statistics are chilling. Almost everybody knows that heart disease is the nation's most deadly affliction, killing more people than any other single cause. The mortality statistics from the office of Population Censuses and Surveys show that more than 100,000 people die each year from heart attack in England and Wales.

Heart disease is usually thought of as a problem that goes with old age, but this is not true. Of course, older people have more heart problems than the young, but heart disease exists in people of all ages. It causes more than one third of all deaths among people under the age of sixty-five. In half a million cases of heart attack, according to a study, more than half of the victims died before they could be brought to hospitals.

Heart disease. That is number one. Following it are the other emergencies that can kill quickly and without warning: choking, stroke, drowning, electric shock, burns, accidents, poisoning, drug overdose, diabetic shock, childbirth.

Preparation by millions of people could cut medical emergency deaths dramatically, some experts believe by as much as half. It doesn't take a great deal of time, money or excessive study, but it does demand that you be willing to learn and read about the various things that can happen in an emergency, and that you be willing to use what you learn. Above all, you must be willing to care and if you are properly armed with the confidence that preparation can supply, it is much easier to care. You can become involved in the welfare of your fellow man.

More than twice as many lives could be saved as are being saved now. Seattle, Washington, proved that it can be done. More than 100,000 people in that city cared enough to learn the basics of saving lives in emergencies, in most cases spending as little as one to four hours in study and practice. The results have been dramatic. More than two and a half times as many life-and-death emergency victims have been saved than before. In other words, for every ten persons saved before the programme was started, twenty-five are being saved now. What a reward for such a small investment in caring!

This book is designed to be the first line of defence in medical emergencies, the weapon to be used by those who witness accidents or who are the first to come on the scene. Later, trained rescue crews and, eventually, doctors will take over, but somebody has to be first. For that first person, this book offers separate, distinct and basic chapters about how to save lives, each chapter complete for fast reference. There need be no fumbling through indexes, no cross-checking, no hunting through wordy chapters looking for the right thing to do, for the treatment that really counts. This means finding the information and putting it to work within seconds, those precious few seconds before somebody dies.

Knowledge and practice can spell instinctive reaction, so there isn't that wasted second when most of us hesitate, frozen in our tracks, waiting for someone else to take over. You must not be shocked into doing nothing, but into doing something.

There is a growing need for participation by everyone in medical emergencies because formally trained personnel simply cannot do it all. We must help them. There are not enough people trained in medicine and first aid to go around in today's world, and there never will be. People are moving faster and doing things that are more dangerous from an illness or accident point of view.

If you are properly armed with the courage born of knowledge, you will be equipped to save a life if you should stumble on a medical emergency. You are there. You see it happen. You know the circumstances of the emergency like nobody else in the world. You see the victim clutch his chest as he falls. You see the swimmer floundering in the depths. But you must know *how* to react in the most effective way, and you must *want* to react. You must care. You cannot walk away, assuming others will take over. This is where the buck must stop – with you. There is need for more participation in emergency care by all of us than ever before, because there are more of us than ever before.

One final point: the life you save could be your own. If you have the knowledge to help others then you are better able to care for yourself in case of injury or sudden illness. If your condition keeps you from treating yourself, then the chances are you will be able to tell others what to do for you.

Joe, the man who had a heart attack on the motorway, was lucky because he had Alma with him and Alma wouldn't give up, even after Joe sank into unconsciousness. She continued to wave at passing traffic until a van stopped. Later she told the ambulance crew, 'They were a scruffy lot, but I love every one of them.' The young people sent the driver of the van racing off for help while they started resuscitation (blowing air into the lungs and helping the heart to pump blood). They did not try to move Joe. Instead they treated him where he lay. Soon Joe was taken to a hospital by ambulance and he recovered.

As Sarah was floating unconscious in the river, Bruce appeared by chance. Also by lucky chance, Bruce had been reading about life-saving only a few days before. He plunged into the river and pulled Sarah to the bank. He cleared sand and weeds from her mouth and then he gave mouth-to-mouth respiration and cardiac compression. He revived Sarah, who was taken to hospital, and she was allowed home, fully recovered, a few days later.

While John, Alison's father-in-law, was slipping into unconsciousness in the restaurant, Alison already was reacting by instinct. She had been studying rescue. Let her tell the story: 'I leaped up and ran round the table, wrapping my arms around Dad from behind. Then I gave him the hard pulls I'd learned about. My husband shouted that some food was coming up, but Dad was still motionless. I just held on and kept thrusting hard until he started breathing again. His colour came back, too. I kept telling myself, First you do this, then you do that, and the steps seemed very logical. I felt strangely calm and confident through it all.' The next day John and his wife drove home on schedule, in good health.

When Fred and Jim opened the door and peered in, they recoiled in surprise and fear. They saw the young woman writhing on the floor and they heard her calls for help. She was beginning to give birth, right now! Fred and Jim, married men and fathers, had read the books. They also were men of courage and common sense. While Fred tried to make the mother-to-be comfortable, Jim phoned the nearest hospital. Help was on the way, but he took instructions from a doctor on the other end of the line, because the baby wasn't going to wait for the ambulance. The men followed the doctor's instructions, but then something went wrong. Half an hour passed, but the baby refused to come out. Only the head was visible. 'Turn the baby's shoulders carefully,' the doctor said, 'but be ready. It may pop straight out when you do.' Fred grinned as he told the story. 'He was right. Out popped the baby, slippery, but we hung on gently. The last we heard, mother and child, a boy, were doing fine. I tell you, attending a birth is quite an experience. There's nothing in the world like it.'

These are true stories and each had a happy ending. Each victim was saved by somebody who was competent, and willing to test that competence. Life is not always like that, but you could make it more of a reality with life-saving knowledge, practice and the courage that comes with these weapons.

Again, these things are what this book is all about. In the pages to come is the information, simple and easy to find. Read carefully and, at the end of each chapter, think about what you would do if you were the central figure in the emergency. We hope you will realize there is something you can do – instantly, instinctively, correctly.

You can save a life.

2. Heart Attack

Heart attacks are the number one killer in England and Wales. They kill over 100,000 people every year. They come in several sizes and degrees of intensity and also from several causes, but all emergency disorders of the heart are called heart attacks. It is true that heart attacks are more likely to happen to older people, but they can strike people of any age.

The effects of these different kinds of heart attacks on their victims may be quite varied, depending on their intensity, but generally you can recognize a heart attack fairly easily. What does a heart attack look like? What does a heart attack feel like? What causes a heart attack? What can you do to help someone having a heart attack?

Here are the answers, put as simply and basically as possible, so that you will be able to do some good if you are there when an attack strikes.

First, you ought to know a little bit about the kinds and causes of heart attacks.

In the classic heart attack, a sudden blocking of the arteries that supply the heart with blood is the cause. It is a result of a slowly developing thickening of the lining of the arteries. This is the condition that causes most heart attacks and the symptoms that go with them.

Angina is a mild form of the same attack. The arteries are only partly blocked. There is some pain, but it is less severe, and usually the attack goes away. Often angina is mistaken for indigestion.

Haemorrhage, shock or drug overdose can cause circulation to fail. The heart may still be beating, but it is so weak that blood is not being circulated.

Cardiac arrest is usually caused by a lack of oxygen in the heart and, as the name implies, the heart stops beating.

Sometimes during heart attacks the heart will beat out of rhythm. Individual muscles beat independently of one another, preventing the heart from doing its pumping job.

Sometimes older people suffer from simple heart failure. The heart is tired and it can no longer carry its normal work load.

Often there are early warning signals in the first stages of a heart attack. It is vital that you recognize them so that you do not waste valuable time deciding if the symptoms are real. Then you can act at once, giving direct aid and taking steps to get professional medical help for the victim. The peak risk of heart attack is in the first moments of the attack. During those moments the victim and those near him are given signals which must be read promptly.

When intense pressure, tightness, or squeezing in the centre of the chest persists for five minutes or more, the warning is clear. If the pain spreads across the chest and possibly to the shoulders, arms, neck or jaw, the warning bells are ringing louder than ever. If this pain is accompanied by sweating, nausea, shortness of breath and faintness, it is imperative that you take immediate action. Serious heart attacks usually result in unconsciousness. The victim's heart may stop beating. He may stop breathing. He will begin to look dead – that is, his skin colour will turn a dead white, grey or grey-blue.

If the victim remains conscious with a beating heart and lungs that breathe – as during an attack of angina – a prompt trip to the hospital is the best thing. Usually ambulances provide self-contained life-support systems and trained personnel to make the trip safer. If there is no professional help available, you must be careful to keep your patient quiet and comfortable. Put him in a semi-sitting posture with feet horizontal. Use pillows or a wall behind him. Wrap him in blankets, jackets or anything else that can help keep him warm.

Then you must decide, if you are alone, whether to leave your patient and go for help or to stay with him. It depends on his condition. If he seems to be holding his own, is breathing well, if his heart has a steady beat and he seems reasonably comfortable, you may decide it's best to go for help. Of course if others are near by, send them. They will do as you say, if you seem to know what you are doing.

If the heart attack is so serious that the patient stops breathing and his heart ceases to beat, then you have your work cut out for you. This is when you must know what to do almost by instinct, so that you do not hesitate. You must move into action at once, in seconds, following basic steps that, with knowledge and practice, can be automatic.

You should know a few things about the heart. It will help your efforts at pumping life back into a victim if you understand what your efforts are for.

All parts of the body require oxygen, but the brain needs more than any other part. The principal function of the heart and lungs is to gather oxygen and pump it throughout the body. Air that comes into the lungs has about 21 per cent oxygen and a trace of carbon dioxide. Air that is exhaled from the lungs has about 16 per cent oxygen and 4 per cent carbon dioxide. This is important.

Your breath contains life-saving oxygen.

The right side of the heart pumps blood to the lungs. There the blood picks up oxygen and releases carbon dioxide as the blood is cleansed. The clean blood, refilled with oxygen, then returns to the left side of the heart. From there it is pumped throughout the body. As the blood travels through the body it releases oxygen and picks up carbon dioxide, after which it flows back to the right side of the heart.

It has been pointed out that the brain needs more oxygen than any other part of the body, and it needs a steady supply. If oxygen is cut off from the body, it is the brain which begins to suffer first. If oxygen-loaded blood is withheld from the brain for only four to six minutes, brain damage begins.

A few minutes without oxygen can kill your patient.

Two things are obvious in all this: breathing lungs and a pumping heart are needed to keep the patient alive; and fast action is vital to get things going and keep them going if you are going to save a life. You can do this without any special equipment. No machines, no oxygen masks, no plastic tubes. Just you, your hands, your lungs, your head – and your heart.

You are at a party, in a car, walking along the street, and you see someone fall to the floor, slump in his seat or plunge to the ground. He is clutching his heart and complaining about the heavy pains that are spreading throughout his upper body. Then he becomes unconscious and his colour turns bad. He is the colour of death. He isn't breathing. He seems dead.

What can you do?

You must get busy *at once* to keep the victim alive. First, take charge. If there are others around, ask them to go for an ambulance and to help you take care of the sick person. If there is only one other person available, make him stay and help you. Your patient may be dying.

Lay the victim on his back, his body flat and on a hard surface. Don't put pillows or anything else under his head to prop it up. If someone else has already done this, take away the things under the head. The head must be on a flat surface and tilted back.

This position of the head is vital to assure that the victim can breathe if his lungs can be made to work. His throat must be clear so that air can pass into his lungs. If the head is lifted or tilted forward, the lower jaw can drop backwards, allowing the tongue to fall back and block the throat. Then the victim may choke to death.

Warning. If the victim has been injured, be wary of moving the head. If you suspect a neck injury, do not move the head, but keep it in a fixed position. The lower jaw can be slid forward by pushing with the fingers at the points of the jaw under the ears. The jaw should be held forward to keep the throat open.

If the neck does not seem to be injured, the head may be safely tilted back. If there is any indication of throat obstruction, you should sweep your fingers into the victim's mouth to make sure breathing is not blocked. In falling, dirt or gravel might have been sucked in. Or he may have vomit or pieces of broken denture in his throat.

To tilt the head, make certain you have the victim on his back, body flat, on a hard surface. A bed is too soft. The floor or level ground is fine. Put one hand under his neck and the other on his forehead. Lift his neck and tilt the head back to extend the neck and lift the tongue out of the throat.

This is the time to *look*, *listen* and *feel* to find out if your patient is breathing. Put your cheek close to his mouth and nose. *Look* at his chest to see if it is rising and falling. *Listen* and *feel* for air moving in and out of the victim. If there is no breathing, you must start artificial respiration at once.

Remember, sending for help, getting the victim on his back on a hard surface, opening his throat and checking for breathing should take only a few seconds. You've got to react quickly, on instinct.

Now it is time for you to breathe life into the victim. He may look dead, but you can't know for sure. So you must get to work. Remember, the brain begins to die after only four to six minutes without oxygen.

Kneel close to the side of the victim's head, leaning over his face. Place a hand under his neck to keep his head tilted back. Put your other hand on his forehead, using the heel to keep his head back and the fingers to reach down over his nose and pinch his nostrils closed.

Open your mouth wide, take a deep breath, and make a tight seal with your lips as you blow into the victim's mouth. Give four quick, full breaths. Don't wait for the victim's chest to fall between the breaths. Give them fast. This pumps a quick first bonus of oxygen into his lungs. You'll know the air is getting into his lungs if you see his chest inflate and then fall. You'll probably feel and hear the air escape from his mouth as he exhales. If your mouth and nose seal are properly tight you'll also feel some resistance as you blow into his mouth. After all, you do need to give enough pressure to lift the chest and inflate the lungs. After the first four quick breaths, you should breathe into the victim's mouth every five seconds, taking your mouth away between breaths so that the victim's lungs can expel the air.

If you can't breathe into the mouth for any reason, such as injury, you can breathe through his nose. If you do this, make certain you keep his mouth closed.

Now it is time to find out if the patient's heart is beating. The best way you can do this is to check for a pulse in his neck. Slip your fingers into the groove between the windpipe and the muscles at the side of the neck. Your touch must be gentle. (Practise by finding your own neck pulse.) This is the best pulse to check because it is the strongest. A pulse may be felt in the neck when none can be felt in the wrist. Also the neck usually is accessible without removing clothing and you already are at the victim's head. You will be wasting less time by checking at the neck. If you can feel no pulse, it means the heartbeat is very weak – or that the heart is not beating at all. *Get going.*

Your patient already has an open throat and you've given him his first breaths of air. *Now you've got to make his heart work.* This also must be done quickly, so that the entire process of placing the victim, opening his throat, giving the first air, checking for a pulse and beginning cardiac compression takes only a few seconds.

Your treatment will be easier, more efficient and more effective from now on if you have help.

Quickly place your helper over the victim's mouth and tell him to blow into the victim's lungs at regular five-second intervals, or once for every five times you push on your patient's chest. Tell him to keep the head back and to hold the nostrils closed, as you did.

You must compress the victim's heart by pressing on his chest with an even rhythm. When you do this properly, you force the heart to pump blood at about one quarter to one third its normal efficiency.

Cardiac compression (heart massage) can work because the heart lies between the breastbone and the tissues above the spine, almost in the centre of the chest. When the lower part of the chest is depressed, the heart's left and right ventricles are squeezed and blood is forced into the large arteries to the lungs, to the brain and to the rest of the body.

Keep your patient horizontal and, remember, no pillows or other cushions may be placed under his head. If he is sitting up there can be no flow of blood to the brain. Make certain he is lying on a hard, flat surface.

Get on your knees, close to the side of the patient's chest. Put the heel of one hand lengthwise on the body, centred over the lower half of the breastbone. Be careful not to place your hand over the lower tip of the breastbone, an area called the xiphoid process. This is too low and the pointed bone could be pressed into internal organs, damaging them. Feel for the tip of the breastbone and measure one and a half inches – about two finger widths – up the centre of the chest. The heel of your hand should be placed just above this point. Put your other hand on top of the first one, keeping your fingers up off the chest so that your pressure is more concentrated.

Then bring your shoulders directly over the victim's chest, keep your arms straight, rock back and forth slightly from the hips and exert pressure vertically downward. This should depress the lower chest one and a half to two inches. Relax after each compression, but keep the heel of your hand on the chest. Allow the chest to return to its normal position after each compression.

You should press down once each second. One way to time your compressions, if you have no watch, is to count, 'One thousand and one, one thousand and two, one thousand and three . . .' and so forth. Each of these counts takes about a second. Remember, your helper should breathe into the patient's mouth every five seconds. There should be no uneven pauses or the victim's blood pressure will drop and there will be no blood flow.

Two rescuers may change positions, if each knows how to perform both cardiac compression and mouth-to-mouth respiration. The switch can be made immediately after the lungs have been filled. The mouth-to-mouth breather must move to your side, place his hands as you lift yours from the chest and continue the cardiac compression with even strokes. You must then move quickly to the victim's mouth to continue the breathing.

If there is no one else around who can or will help, or if you are alone when the victim is stricken, you're going to have to work much harder. You must move back and forth between the victim's mouth and chest. The chest must be compressed faster, about eighty times a minute. This can be timed by counting,

'One thousand, two thousand, three thousand . . .' and so forth, so that the counting is about twenty-five per cent faster than with two rescuers.

After every series of fifteen cardiac compressions, you must hurry to the victim's mouth and give two fast and full breaths. Then get back to his chest and give fifteen more cardiac compressions.

The techniques for infants and children up to five or six years old are much the same, except that breaths and cardiac compression should be given faster and more gently. A child's body is smaller, of course, and softer. A child's heart lies slightly higher in his chest, and you should apply pressure in the middle of the breastbone. For infants, you should use only the tips of your middle and index fingers. For small children, use the heel of one hand only. The small chest is more pliable than the chest of an adult, so be very gentle. The heart should be compressed eighty to one hundred times a minute. Give one breath for each five heart pumps. Infants and small children should have a firm support beneath the upper back. Your hand or a folded blanket will do. This is because a child's windpipe is softer and more flexible than an adult's. Lifting the back helps keep the head tilted back, keeping the windpipe straight and open.

If you are treating an infant or child by yourself, compress his heart at the same faster rate and give two quick breaths into his lungs after each fifteen heart compressions.

After the first minute of mouth-to-mouth breathing and cardiac compression you should very quickly check your patient's neck pulse for signs of a beating heart. If you have a helper who is breathing into the patient's mouth, he may check the patient's eye pupils occasionally to see if they react to light. If the pupils grow smaller in the light, this is good. It means the brain still has oxygen and blood. If the pupils do not react to light this is bad. However, the neck pulse is a more reliable sign of life than pupils. The breather also should *watch* for signs that the chest is rising and falling on its own, and *feel* and *listen* for air being taken into and carried out of the lungs.

In rare cases, your patient may have had a tracheotomy, so that he breathes through a hole in his throat. If the victim does breathe in this way, you should give him air directly through the neck hole, ignoring his nose and mouth.

Here are a few final words of advice:
Resuscitation (mouth-to-mouth assisted breathing and cardiac compression) should be started in cases of sudden, unexpected death. If you're not sure, start resuscitation at once anyway. *Don't waste time.* Don't make a prolonged examination of the victim. Don't take time to go for distant assistance. Don't bother removing clothing. Don't move him unnecessarily. *Get going.*

If you are able to keep your patient alive, even if he seems much better after a while, remember that he should be taken to expert care as fast as possible. If he is improved, make him warm and comfortable when resuscitation is no longer needed. Then see that he gets to a hospital. You may have sent for help already.

Perhaps you can flag down a passing car, or anyone who is willing to help. If there is no one else, it's up to you to determine whether you can safely leave your patient and go for help.

Finally, even if you have done everything by the book, but an hour has gone by and your patient shows no signs of life, it means you were not successful. If the patient dies after you have done your best, do not blame yourself or be discouraged from trying to help someone else in the future. There are no guarantees of success when it is a matter of life and death. You cared enough to try and you should never stop caring. That is important.

Artificial respiration is a life-saving skill that is difficult to learn perfectly by reading about it. You can actually practise on models by taking a course at your local Red Cross or St John's Ambulance Association.

Heart Attack

What to look for

Severe pain – centre of chest.

Pressure and pain continue.
Pain spreads to shoulders, arms,
neck, jaw.

Intense pain continues. Skin
goes dead white, bluish or grey.
Victim sweats.

Patient unconscious

Breathing stops

No heartbeat apparent

Two-person resuscitation

What to do

If you suspect a heart attack
call a doctor. Try to calm and
reassure patient.

Lay patient in semi-sitting
position. Keep patient warm. If
alone, make decision now to
stay or go for help.

Phone for emergency
ambulance. Reassure patient
that help is coming.

Take action
Lay patient flat on back (no
pillow). Tilt head back. Clear
throat if necessary. Check for
breathing.

Start mouth-to-mouth respiration
Kneel close to head. Hand
under neck. Pinch nostrils shut.
**Blow 4 quick, full breaths
into patient's mouth**. Check
pulse – if present. Breathe into
mouth every 5 seconds.

Start chest compressions

Rate of 60 chest compressions
a minute, regular, smooth, even,
without interruptions. Rate of
one breath between every 5
compressions.

One-person resuscitation	Rate of 80 chest compressions per minute, regular, smooth, even, without interruptions. Rate of 2 quick breaths within 5 seconds between each series of 15 compressions.
	Check neck pulse after one minute and every few minutes thereafter.
If heartbeat returns	Assist respiration, continue to monitor pulse.
	Continue resuscitation until help arrives.

Action sequence for resuscitation

1. Lay patient flat on back.

2. **Open throat by tilting head back.**

3. Look, listen and feel for breathing.

4. **If no breathing, give 4 short, hard breaths.**

5. Check for neck pulse. If no pulse, **begin resuscitation at once.**

6. **Two-person resuscitation**
   Rate of 60 chest compressions a minute, regular, smooth, even, without interruptions. Rate of one breath between every 5 compressions.

7. **One-person resuscitation**
   Rate of 80 chest compressions per minute, regular, smooth, even, without interruptions. Rate of 2 quick breaths within 5 seconds between each series of 15 compressions.

8. Check pulse at neck and examine eye pupils to determine if resuscitation is effective. **Keep going**.

9. **Continue as long as possible, until help arrives or pulse resumes**.

Xs show the major pulse points of the body – places where the pulse is most easily felt because the artery is close to the skin and located directly over a bone. The pulse is a bumping that is felt when a finger is placed over an artery.

In the frontal view, from the top, are the following pulse points: carotid, brachial, radial, femoral and posterior tibial. In the side view, from the top, are the following pulse points: temporal, carotid and popliteal.

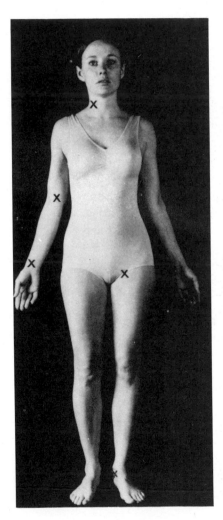
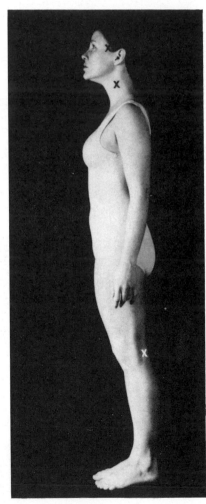

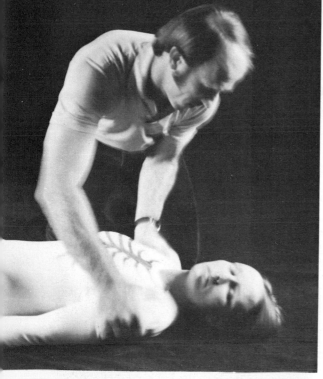

The first step with an unconscious person is to 'shake and shout'. Grasp shoulders as shown and shake vigorously while shouting at the same time. Consciousness may return.

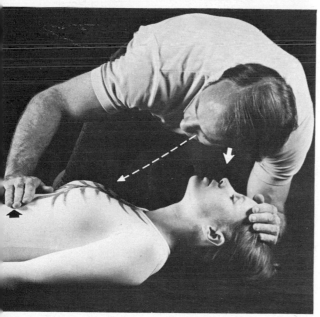

To find out if your patient is breathing, *look, listen* and *feel.* Look to see if the chest is rising and falling, listen for the sound of air, get close to feel if there is air on your face.

No pulse and no breathing indicate that the heart has stopped and resuscitation must begin immediately to restore blood circulation. Pupils begin to dilate (as above) within a minute after the heart stops. If resuscitation treatment is successful, the pupils will contract to normal size.

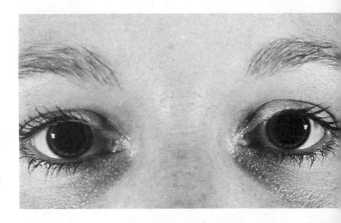

Tilt the victim's head back with your hands on forehead and back of the neck to help open airway.

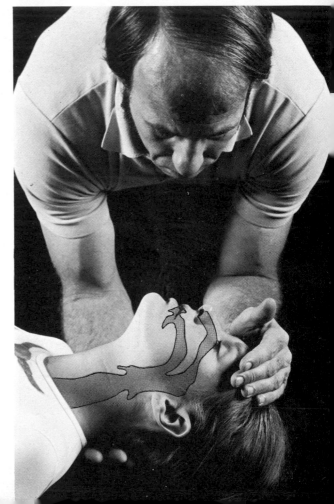

Make certain your first breath of air is a big one. Fill your lungs with fresh air before you begin to breathe life into your patient.

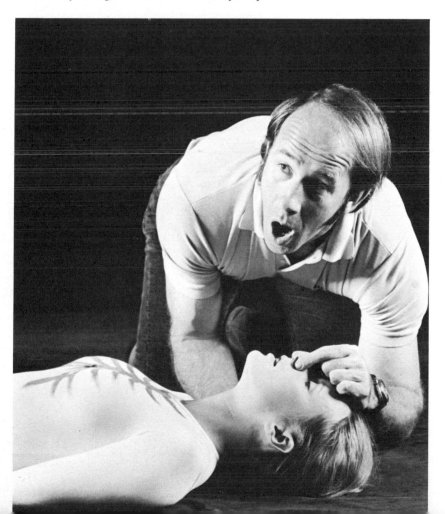

Keep the head tilted
back, pinch the nostrils
closed and make a tight
seal with your mouth
on the victim's mouth.
Breathe four quick, full
breaths into the victim.
Allow your patient to
exhale naturally and
then continue with one
breath every five
seconds.

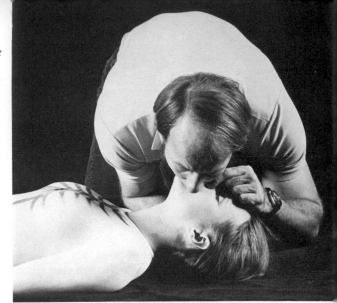

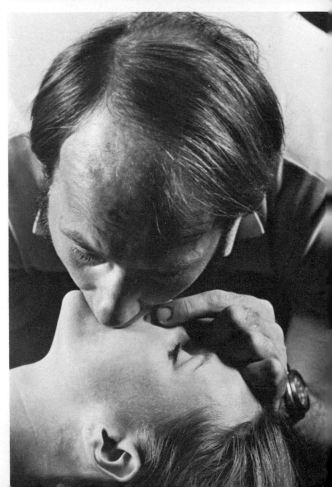

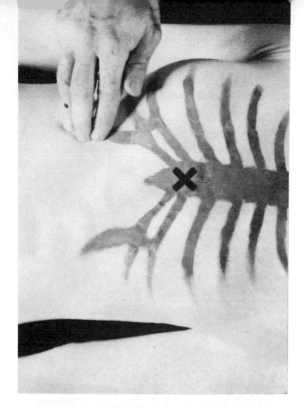

To locate the proper place to use your hands, arms and shoulders for cardiac compression, begin by tracing the lower edge of the rib-cage as shown.

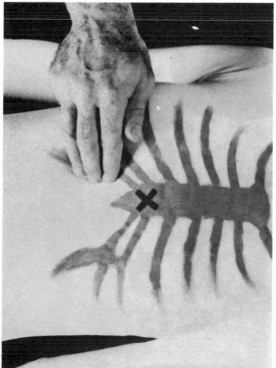

Continue to move your fingers gently along the rib bone. This will lead you to the tip of the breastbone.

The X in the photographs shows the lower limit for the hand during cardiac compression. Avoid the tip of the breastbone below this point.

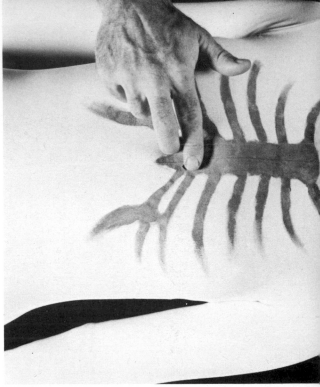

The heel of your hand must be used to exert pressure on the chest and, thus, the heart. Use your other hand to hold the fingers back, so that the pressure point is as limited as possible.

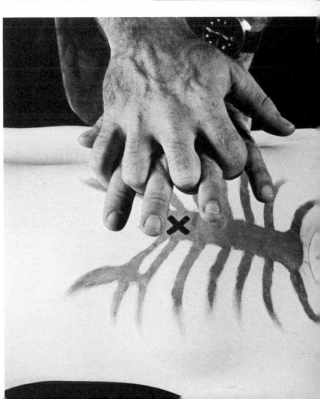

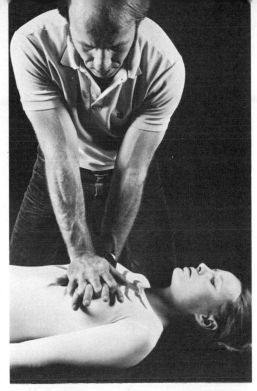

The rescuer keeps his arms straight as he swings the weight of his body over the victim and exerts strong pressure straight down. Use your body's weight, not just your arm muscles.

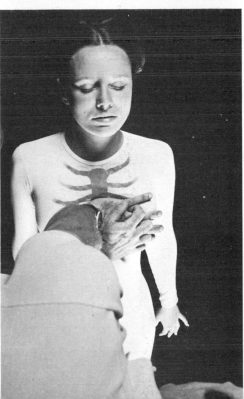

View from above showing how the downward pressure of the hands, arms and shoulders is used. Pressure should be firm, regular and applied once per second.

Multiple exposure shows how to move from mouth-to-mouth ventilation to chest-heart compressions. Give fifteen compressions (see text), then quickly move back to mouth and give two fast but full breaths. Continue with fifteen thrusts to every two breaths.

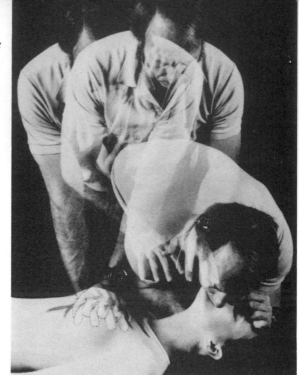

Use a helper if you possibly can to give one quick breath after every fifth compression while you compress the victim's heart at the rate of one compression per second. It is a two-person non-stop operation and is the best way to get the heart and lungs working again.

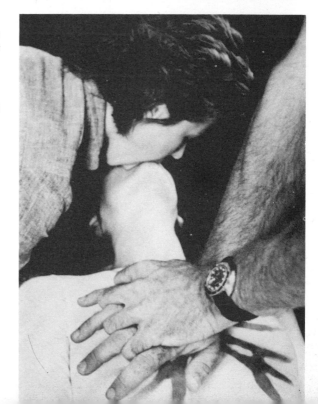

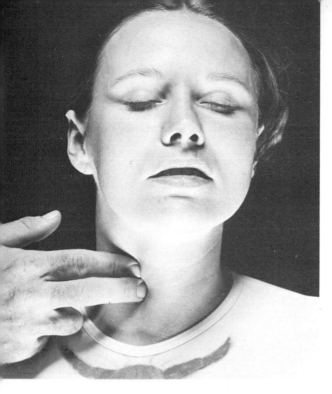

The neck carotid pulse is the most reliable. Find it by sliding your fingers into the groove between the trachea and the muscles at the side of the neck. Check the pulse to see how you're doing.

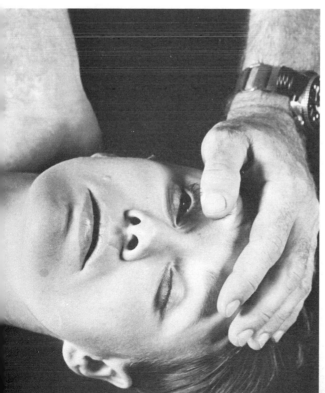

The pupils of the eye should be checked to see if they have become smaller. This is the best way to find out if oxygenated blood is being delivered to the victim's brain.

3. Choking

Few medical emergencies are more bizarre than choking. Often the setting for tragedy is light-hearted and gay. Many choking accidents take place at parties, where there are lots of people about, where there is laughter and where there is alcohol.

No one is safe from choking. This accident can happen to anybody. This is more true of choking than such emergencies as heart attack, stroke, diabetic shock or drug overdose, which usually happen because of age, ill health or indulgence. You can be any age, in perfect health and a person who avoids dangerous habits – the threat of death from choking is still present.

Choking ranks seventh in England and Wales as a cause of accidental death. Experts estimate that choking takes four to five hundred lives every year. Among choking victims are those who are young and old, rich and poor, alone and with friends. Many chokings, those with happy endings as well as those which end with a victim being covered with a white sheet, involve accidents with food. Thus the term 'café coronary' was born because witnesses often mistake choking symptoms for heart attacks.

One evening in 1956 a man ate a heavy Sunday meal at his home. Later, not feeling well, he went to bed. Sometime in the night he became nauseated. The next morning he was found dead in his bed, a victim of choking on food that had come up from his stomach. Out of sight and hearing of others, the victim had been unable to help himself. A musical genius and the sounds of a sweet trombone died with that man. He was Tommy Dorsey.

Irony marked the death of the US wire service bureau chief Joe Brooks, who choked to death in a restaurant in 1974. In his reporting at the capital city of his state he wrote an article about a Bill covering emergency action that could be taken by restaurant personnel when a patron is choking on food. Two weeks later Brooks himself became a choking victim. Public education and action came along too late to help him.

A political campaigner was in his plane, weary from weeks of travelling thousands of miles to face voters. Eating casually, his mind on other matters, the man suddenly choked. He gasped and looked about in panic. He was lucky, for there were competent people close by, and an aide grasped the victim about the abdomen and thrust hard into his middle. The deadly bit of food came up in a few seconds and the victim was all right after he caught his breath. The culprit was an unchewed peanut. No, the victim wasn't Jimmy Carter. It was Ronald Reagan.

The telephone rang at a police station. A seventeen-year-old girl was frantic. Her grandmother was choking on a piece of food. 'We need an ambulance,' the girl wailed. The constable, who had been studying life-saving techniques, immediately sent an ambulance on its way, but he also had the good sense to keep the girl on the telephone. Yes, there was another person in the house other than the seventy-nine-year-old grandmother – the girl's older brother. The constable relayed instructions to the brother through the girl and, although the grandmother actually had stopped breathing for several seconds, her grandson cleared her throat and saved her life. Later the constable sent a bouquet of roses to the hospital where the grandmother had been taken for observation.

There *are* effective ways to help choking victims, ways that work most of the time. Speed in rescue is as important in bringing aid to chokers as it is to victims of heart attack. Often the results are much more dramatic, because while heart-attack victims usually remain weak and ill after the rescue, victims of choking usually are feeling much better moments after effective treatment.

The effectiveness of choking rescue techniques has been studied and tested by a number of medical teams using animals and volunteer humans. Rescue, properly carried out, worked successfully 97 per cent of the time. The volunteers were actually permitted to choke on pieces of meat which were tethered with string just in case.

Dr Henry J. Heimlich, the Cincinnati surgeon who devised a choking rescue technique which bears his name, has received many hundreds of newspaper clippings, health department reports and thank-you notes over the years. Dr Heimlich knows of at least 750 choking victims who owe their lives to rescuers who used his technique. These include two eight-year-olds who saved younger children and twenty-six quick-thinking victims who actually saved themselves.

Two doctors studied the food choking problem for years and they have come up with some useful observations. Victims are usually careless. They have often been drinking, and their food has not been properly chewed. Often older victims wear dentures, which make choking more of a hazard because the food is not chewed as easily as with natural teeth.

The most common causes of choking on food are:
- large, poorly chewed pieces of meat
- laughing and being otherwise distracted when there is food in the mouth
- moderate to heavy drinking of alcohol while eating
- upper and lower dentures.

There are reasonably precise ways to tell a choking victim from a heart-attack victim. There are ways to help these victims and, as has been shown, these ways are remarkably effective. Often both victim and rescuer walk away from the scene before the arrival of official rescue teams and, therefore, they do not become part of our statistical records.

Many times a rescuer must work alone, even when there are others present. A medical emergency does not prompt bystanders to action if they are not prepared through knowledge, training, common sense and – most of all – caring. If you care you can help, even if you must do the job alone. As one ambulance-man said, 'You can't count on other people helping you, especially if you're in a restaurant among strangers.'

There are ways to avoid choking by food or by foreign substances.

• Food should always be cut into small pieces and be chewed slowly and thoroughly, especially by people wearing dentures.

• Avoid laughing and talking during chewing and swallowing. Avoid excessive drinking of alcohol just before and during meals.

• Don't let children run or play while they have food or other things in their mouths. Keep dangerous things such as marbles, beads, drawing-pins and rings from drink cans out of the reach of infants and small children.

What does all this mean to you? The answer should be obvious. You can learn to recognize a choking victim. You can learn how to use precise steps to deal with the emergency. You can take charge when others are afraid, unwilling or too uninformed to know what to do.

Rescuing a choking victim

There are varying degrees of choking and it is important that you distinguish them from other emergencies so that you will be able to give the right treatment. You must be careful not to confuse choking victims with victims of fainting, stroke, heart attack or other conditions that cause breathing problems or unconsciousness.

Often the choking victim is only partly cut off from normal breathing. In other words, he may be able to breathe reasonably well by himself. In these cases the victim is able to cough, but frequently there is a wheezing sound between coughs. As long as the victim is able to speak, breathe, cough and make efforts to help himself, *do not* interfere with his efforts. Don't slap him, hug him or anything else. Keep your hands off.

His breathing may deteriorate, however. You can tell this by a cough that becomes weak and ineffective. He may make high-pitched noises while trying to breathe, a crowing sound. If his breathing comes very close to stopping, you should be able to see his colour change – to a dead white, grey, blue or grey-green.

You can be pretty sure the victim is unable to breathe at all when he is unable to speak or cough. Often, either as a natural gesture or as a result of training (it's the recognized distress signal for choking), the victim will clutch his throat with his thumb and fingers. If you shout at him 'Can you speak?' and the victim cannot answer, it's time for prompt action.

As in the case of heart attack, fast action is essential. You don't have time to go for help. Send someone else to the telephone or to the street to call for assistance. You've got to get to work immediately.

If you can't get air into the victim within four to six minutes, he will begin to die.

Suppose the victim is unconscious and you are not given the telltale distress clues – the hand at the throat, the wheezing and crowing, the obvious distress signals of a person unable to breathe.

You must check to see if his throat is blocked by trying to ventilate him, by trying to force air from your own lungs into his. Use the method explained in the chapter on heart attacks. Place the victim on his back, flat on the floor or the ground. Remember, no pillows or anything else propping up his head. Tilt the head back and place one hand under the neck and the other on the forehead. Pinch his nostrils closed. Seal your mouth over the victim's open mouth and blow in, hard. Watch to see if the victim's chest rises.

If you can't make the victim's chest rise by forcing air into his body, the throat is blocked. *The victim is choking.*

Once again, speed is essential and you will have better chances of success if you can start helping a choking victim before he loses consciousness. *Every second counts.* You've got to get the obstruction out of his throat so that he can breathe again, on his own, before his body is damaged by a lack of oxygen.

The conscious victim

First, let's help a person who is choking but who is still conscious. There are two things for you to do:

- Strike him sharply on the back.
- Press your fist into his abdomen in a quick upward thrust.

Now we will show you how to do these things most effectively.

If a person is choking and his breathing blocked but he is still conscious, it probably means you were there when it happened. It doesn't take long for a person who cannot breathe to lose consciousness.

You must shout at him, 'Can you speak?' If his only response is to stagger, turn pale and clutch at his throat, go to work. Remember, if he is able to speak, to cough, to make rasping noises as though he is painfully drawing in air, don't interfere with him. It's better to let him try to cough it up himself.

But, if he cannot speak or cough and is apparently unable to breathe at all, then you know you must go to work at once.

• Strike him sharply on the back. If he is standing or sitting, you must stand slightly behind and to one side of him. Then strike him with the heel of your hand, right between the shoulder blades. Do it quickly, forcefully and in rapid succession, *four* times. Don't just pat him. They must be hard blows.

If the victim is lying down, get down on your knees and roll him to his side, facing you, with his chest against your knees. Then give him the same series of four sharp blows with the heel of your hand, again between his shoulder blades.

If the victim does not respond, if he continues to clutch his throat, turn a bad colour and to stagger in obvious distress, you must continue.

• Give him *four* quick abdominal thrusts. If the victim is standing or sitting, stand behind him and wrap your arms around his waist. Put the thumb side of your fist against his abdomen, slightly above the navel and below the ribs. Grasp your fist with your other hand and press it into the victim's abdomen with a quick, upward thrust. Remember, the thumb of your fist hand should be on the inside pressing into the abdomen.

If the conscious victim is lying down, place him on his back and kneel beside him. Place the heel of one hand in the middle of his abdomen, in the same spot you would if he were sitting or standing. Place your other hand on top of the first and stiffen your arms. Then rock forward and give that same quick upward thrust towards the chest. Do this *four* times, firmly and sharply.

Whether the victim is standing, sitting or lying down, give these four thrusts quickly, in rapid succession. Be careful, but make the thrusts firm and sharp.

Repeat the blows on his back and the abdominal thrusts as long as necessary, either until he coughs up the thing that was blocking his throat or until he loses consciousness. If you see anything in his mouth or upper throat, pull it out.

The unconscious victim

If the victim becomes unconscious despite your efforts, your job becomes more difficult. Now it's a race with death. Remember, you have only a few minutes to get air into him before he begins to die.

If the victim is not breathing but you can breathe for him – that is, his throat *is not blocked* – begin mouth-to-mouth respiration immediately. If there is no pulse, give him cardiac compression as well, in the way explained in the chapter on heart attacks.

Whenever you see foreign matter in his mouth, remove it with your fingers, if you can. Otherwise, treat the victim as you would the victim of a heart attack.

If the victim is unconscious and you cannot breathe for him – that is, if his throat *is blocked* so that you can't force air into his lungs – roll him against you, his chest against your knees.

Slap him sharply on the back, four times, exactly the way you would for a conscious victim who is lying down.

Then shift the victim to his back and give him four quick and forceful manual abdominal thrusts, again in the same way you would if he were conscious and lying down.

Then probe in his mouth for foreign objects. You might have successfully moved something up from the throat into the mouth, or at least higher in the throat so that you can grasp it or hook it out.

To probe with your fingers, place the victim on his back. Grasp his tongue and lower jaw with your thumb and fingers and lift. This draws his tongue away from the back of his throat and away from anything that might be lodged there. This alone could help to relieve part of the obstruction.

Now, with your other hand, insert your index finger down the inside of his cheek and deeply into his throat to the base of his tongue. Then use a hooking motion to dislodge the object and work it up into his mouth so that you can grasp it with your fingers. Be careful not to press the object deeper into the throat.

You have done four things for the unconscious victim.
- You tried to force air into his lungs with your own breath.
- You slapped him sharply on the back, four times.
- You knelt beside him and thrust into his abdomen, four times.
- You probed his throat in hopes of removing the blocking object.

This is the correct procedure, and you must keep doing these four things in the same sequence. If during your rescue attempt you are successful in removing the object from his throat, give him mouth-to-mouth respiration if he remains unconscious. If his pulse stops, you must also give him cardiac compression. Do not waste time, however, attempting chest compression until adequate ventilation is established.

Remember to persist. Keep trying, just as you would for the victim of a heart attack. As the victim becomes more deprived of air his muscles will relax and the manoeuvres that did not work earlier may begin to do the job.

When the muscles relax or an object is partially dislodged in the throat so that the air passage is partly open, slow, full and forceful ventilation may help to keep a victim alive.

Any time there is vomit or any other matter in his mouth or throat, turn his head to the side and wipe the material out as best you can. Then proceed with the sequence of rescue steps. *Keep trying*.

There are a few exceptions to these rescue techniques. Here they are.

Suppose the victim is so fat around the middle that you can't get your arms around him. Or suppose the victim is pregnant and you cannot press against her abdomen without danger of harming mother and unborn child.

An alternative technique to the abdominal thrust is the chest thrust. If the victim is sitting or standing, stand behind him and place your clenched fist and other hand on his breastbone, up in the middle, not over the rib-cage or the fragile tip of the breastbone. Then thrust in the usual manner. If the victim is lying down, kneel beside his body and place the heel of your hand over the centre of the breastbone, the same as for cardiac compression. Deliver the four chest thrusts sharply.

If the victim is an infant or small child, you must be more gentle with your slapping and thrusting. The child may be picked up for the careful chest thrusts. Also, a small child may be placed face down along your forearm while you slap its back. Keeping its head low may help dislodge whatever is blocking its throat.

Finally, if you should happen to choke when you are alone, you can help yourself. Press your own fist and other hand into your abdomen in the way described for the standing victim. Or you may lean forward to press your abdomen over any solid object, such as the back of a chair, the edge of a sink or a porch railing. The object pressing into your body may help to force out the thing blocking your throat. But remember, you must think and move fast.

Once again, persist in your efforts to help the choking victim. If you have the strength born of confidence, knowledge and caring, you will give him your best efforts. If you fail, try not to be discouraged and, most certainly don't feel you should neglect a later opportunity to save someone else.

Obviously, in your back-slapping and your abdomen-thrusting you are trying to force a sudden rush of air up the victim's windpipe to eject the thing blocking his throat.

This has been compared to the pressure in a bottle of champagne which pushes out the cork with explosive force.

It's an apt comparison. If you are successful, it's an occasion for champagne.

Choking

What to look for	What to do
Victim gasps, clutches throat. Breathing difficult, looks panicky.	Be alerted – watch closely, and be prepared to assist.
Patient has difficulty coughing. Makes wheezing sounds.	Step in and prepare to help if victim obviously cannot help himself.
Victim has difficulty speaking, difficulty being understood.	Shout at victim, 'Can you speak? Can you cough it up?'

Victim's breath close to stopping; appears unable to answer or cough

If conscious	**Take action**
If victim is standing	Strike sharply on back 4 times. Press fist into abdomen 4 times.
If victim is lying down	Get on your knees. Roll victim on side. Bring victim's chest against your knees and deliver: 4 sharp blows with heel of your hand between shoulder blades; 4 quick abdominal thrusts. Repeat blows and thrusts as needed until successful or patient unconscious.

If unconscious

4-step sequence
- Attempt to blow air into lungs.
- Slap back sharply 4 times.
- Abdominal thrusts 4 times.
- Probe mouth for blockages.

If victim continues unconscious — Repeat 4-step sequence above.

As victim is deprived of air, muscles will relax and blocking material may be easier to remove.

Don't give up. Continue efforts.

When successful in removing obstruction

Give 4 quick full breaths. Check pulse. Start resuscitation if necessary.

If victim is infant or child

Be more gentle with slapping and thrusting.

If victim is very fat or pregnant

Use chest thrust instead of abdominal thrust.

If victim is yourself

If alone, press fist into abdomen. Press abdomen over back of chair, edge of sink, railing. Force fingers down throat, regurgitate.

Action sequence for choking victim

If victim is conscious	4 sharp blows in the middle of back. 4 strong abdominal thrusts.
If victim is lying down	Kneel. Roll victim on side up against your knees and strike 4 sharp blows with heel of your hand between shoulder blades.
	Kneel beside victim and use heel of hand for 4 sharp abdominal thrusts.

If victim is unconscious	Try to ventilate him.
	4 sharp blows to the back.
	4 deep abdominal thrusts.
	Probe mouth for blocking matter. Remove.
If victim does not respond	**Do not give up. Keep repeating this 4-step sequence.**
If victim is fat or pregnant	Use chest thrusts instead of abdominal thrusts.
Infants and small children	Infants may be held feet high, head low and face down along your forearm as you slap.
If you are choking and alone	Use your two fists for abdominal thrusts. Bend over back of chair, over edge of sink, railing, etc. Exert hard and repeated pressure to force blocking object up. Push fingers deep down throat to regurgitate.

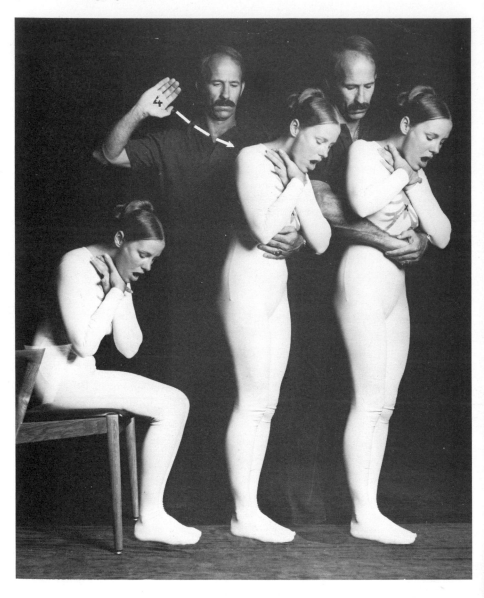

Your victim is choking. You must act fast. If she can cough on her own, leave her alone. If not, deliver four quick firm blows between the shoulder blades. Then apply four abdominal thrusts.

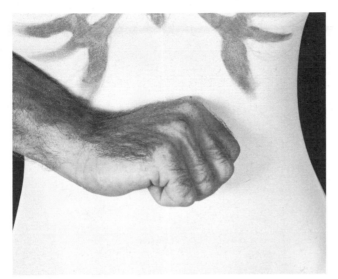

Find the proper place to position your hand, midway between the lower end of the breastbone and the navel. Use your thumb side as you place the first hand in the proper position. Work fast.

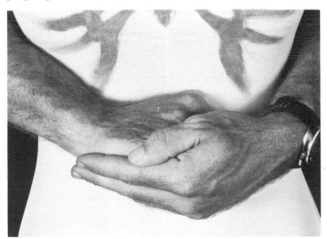

Here you see the correct position for both hands. Now you are ready to deliver an abdominal thrust. The object is to force a quick burst of air up through the throat to dislodge an obstruction.

If the victim is sitting
down, you can still
deliver the four quick
back blows and then go
on to the other steps
towards relieving her of
the obstruction. You
must act in seconds.

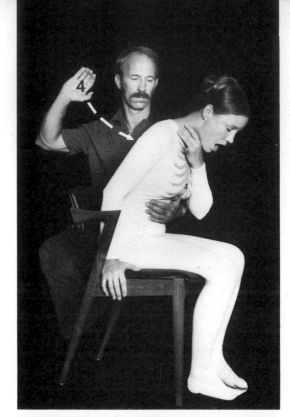

This shows how you
can deliver the
abdominal thrust with
your victim sitting
down. If she collapses
and loses
consciousness, you
must work towards
opening an airway as
fast as you can.

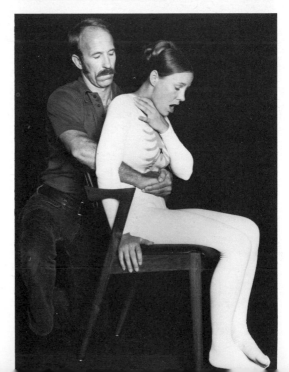

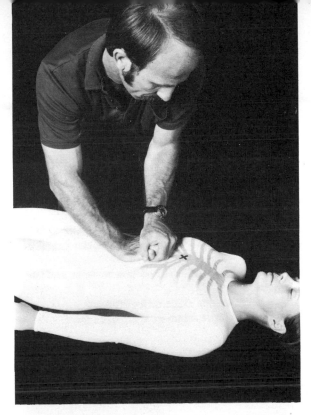

An effective abdominal thrust to clear the throat of a choking victim is achieved by placing your clenched hands in the upper abdomen between the lower end of the breastbone and the navel as shown. Deliver four firm thrusts.

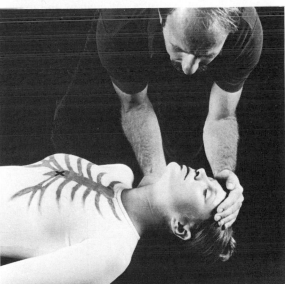

Clear the victim's throat through back blows and/or abdominal thrusts. Only after clearing the throat and getting air into the lungs should you begin artificial respiration and cardiac compression, if necessary. See pages 20–22.

4. Drowning

The tragedy of drowning is that it happens so often when the cause is simple carelessness. Nowhere in the process of saving a life is the principle of *safety first* so obvious. A little preparation, a little caution, a little common sense are all that is needed to prevent thousands of drowning deaths a year. More than 400 people drown each year in England and Wales, and most of them didn't even intend to get wet.

Two thirds of the nation's drowning victims don't know how to swim, and half of the victims are alone at the time.

How much grief could be avoided if simple rules were observed:

- If you're going near water, learn how to swim.
- Don't go in or on the water alone.
- Don't get careless in or near water.
- Learn a few basic rescue techniques to help get victims (including yourself) out of the water.
- Learn how to treat them after you've brought them ashore.

Even non-swimmers can help rescue victims in deep water. Literally extending a helping hand may do the job. Or keeping calm and helping to calm a struggling victim. Or simply throwing him something to hang on to.

Anybody can drown. It's a fact. Strong swimmers and divers have been known to go under the surface for no known reason. Perhaps a muscle spasm, a sudden attack of illness, a psychological quirk that terrorizes them for some mysterious reason. Overconfidence is a deadly enemy for swimmers. Nobody knows for sure. Anybody can drown, but some groups of people are more at risk.

A medical director of a children's hospital who has studied drowning cases has found that the drowning victim is most often a boy under the age of five, and he is most likely to drown between 1 and 3 p.m. on a weekday within fifty yards of his own house. But drowning victims do come in all sizes, ages, colours and both sexes.

'Almost invariably, the children were not observed to be drowning,' the medical director said. 'The adults were not there. The children were discovered missing. Often the children were able to swim. I am concerned about the false sense of security that a parent might have if he thinks his child is water-safe.' An interesting observation, one that all parents ought to think about.

The boy didn't think himself much of a hero, but the Boy Scouts presented the fourteen-year-old lad with their highest award for heroism. It happened during a summer afternoon when he was walking past the family swimming pool. 'I saw him, my cousin, lying in the bottom of the pool,' the boy said. 'I just jumped in and pulled him out. He'd probably be dead if I hadn't walked past when I did.' True enough, for haste in rescue is as important for those threatened with drowning as it is for choking and heart-attack victims. The young hero's father rushed to the side of the pool and gave the three-year-old cousin artificial respiration until he was breathing on his own again.

The young couple were on their honeymoon, and the bridegroom couldn't resist showing his pretty young wife his skill on the high diving board. But something went wrong. The young man slipped and his head hit a lower board on the way down. He plunged into the pool like something dead, but his quick-thinking bride plunged after him from the side of the pool. Seeing the pink tinge of blood in the water from a wound, she carefully lifted her husband to the surface. There she called for help, rather than try to pull him from the water herself. The other rescuers saw the blood, and they managed to remove the young man from the pool with a minimum of twisting and turning of his head and body. He was saved from drowning and also from possibly being crippled for life because of an abused broken neck or back.

Precautions which should be taken

Swimmer and boater, beware. You are neither as strong nor as skilled in or on the water as you think you are. You shouldn't swim or go out in a boat alone. You shouldn't allow yourself to become so tired that your body is weakened or your mind is apt to become careless. There are several organizations that will teach you to swim. They can also teach you safety-first in the water and in a boat.

There should be rescue equipment, preferably life jackets of some sort, for each person in a small boat. The jacket should be *worn*, not simply left lying about somewhere half forgotten and out of reach. A small boat can be upset quite easily at any time, even in the placid waters of a lake. Small boats are more dangerous, of course, where the water is rougher.

Despite the obvious fact that simple common sense can prevent most drownings, it has been shown that many people do not bother to use common sense – especially if they're with a group of friends and having a good time.

So it is quite possible that one day a person in danger of drowning will desperately need your help. It's up to you to prepare yourself for rescue as best you can. Also, there is a bonus in it for you. Your *own* life will be safer because you'll have learned to be safety-conscious and you'll have learned techniques that you can apply to your own survival in case something should happen.

The conscious victim

In open water

You are on the beach, or near the edge of a pool, or on the quayside, and someone in the water gets into trouble. There are several ways you can help, even without any special rescue equipment.

Lying flat on the pier or by the edge of the pool and reaching an arm towards the victim is one of the safest ways of giving assistance. In this way you are able to reach further over the water, and you are stabilized by lying down so that a frantic victim is less likely to pull you into the water.

Sometimes a victim can be talked out of his panic and helped to find his footing and the way towards the shore. The proper thing to do depends on the situation, of course, and you must use your best judgement.

If the victim is out of reach, in deep water, and you can't swim, you have no choice but to encourage him and to look for life-saving devices to thrust at him: poles, life-belts, empty plastic bottles with watertight tops, rope, anything that can support the victim's weight.

The rescuer, whether he can swim or not, should be careful not to let a panicky victim grab him. A drowning man or woman can have unreasoning, deadly strength. All too often the result is two drowning victims instead of one.

If you are swimming or wading to a victim, keep your eyes on him as you approach to see how rational he seems to be. If you have equipment, something that floats, keep it between yourself and the victim, so that you and he can hold opposite sides. Try to keep him calm by talking to him. Once the victim grasps the floating device, start pulling him slowly towards the shore. If the victim panics and climbs across the device towards you, let go and move away.

Do not let a panicky victim grab you. Do not try a swimming rescue of a conscious victim unless you are specially trained in life-saving.

Ice

Rescuing someone who has fallen through ice is more dangerous and difficult than a rescue in open water. The ice may break again, trapping the rescuer. All the while haste is necessary because a person can live only a few minutes in freezing water.

Be wary of ice over water. Ice clouded with air bubbles should be avoided; it is usually weak. Do not go near partially submerged obstacles such as stumps or rocks; the ice is likely to be weaker there. Ice moving over water is likely to be unsafe. Ice should be studied for man-made hazards before it is walked on, skated on or skied on – things like places where holes have been cut, where ice has been broken, and so forth. Such areas should be marked as dangerous to warn others.

When you try to rescue someone who has fallen through ice you must be careful to protect yourself. Anything that helps you distribute your weight over a wide area of ice will increase your own safety. If you lie prone on the ice and keep your arms and legs spread wide as you approach the victim, you'll be less likely to break through.

A light ladder fourteen to eighteen feet long is valuable. A rope can be tied on to one end and it can then be shoved out on the ice for the victim to grasp. If a rescuer must go with the ladder, the length helps distribute his weight. If the end of the ladder breaks through the ice, it can be pulled back to shore by others on the end of the rope.

Other ice rescue devices include floating things that can be pushed or thrown to the victim and even a human chain of rescuers linked at hands and feet, prone on the ice.

Getting back into your boat

When you are climbing into a small boat, you should remember two fundamental things: *keep low* and *distribute your weight* carefully. Always step into a boat somewhere near the middle and try to place your weight as near to the centre as possible. Don't stand up in a small boat. Drop to your knees and sit down. That's keeping low so that you will be less likely to capsize the craft.

It's a good idea to practise getting into a capsized boat. You should do this if you are going out in a rowing boat or canoe for the first time, or if the quirks of the craft are unfamiliar to you.

Let's suppose you are somehow thrown from a small boat which has not capsized. It's floating high and relatively dry next to you. Reach over the side amidships, placing your hands on the bottom of the boat as close to the middle as you can. Press down with your hands and kick your feet to the surface of the water. Still pressing down, kick your feet until the boat slides under your body. You're trying to raise your body, depress the boat and at the same time pull the boat under yourself. Keep your head low, and when it is against the far side of the boat, roll over and sit down in the bottom.

Suppose your boat is swamped as you fall out. You get back into your swamped boat in the same manner, keeping your weight as low as you can by rolling over to sit down once you're in the middle. Then you can paddle or row towards the shore, using only your hands, if necessary, whether the boat is swamped or not.

Canoes and rowing boats almost always float if capsized or filled with water, so remember always to stay close to your boat if you're far from shore. You're safer clinging to the boat than attempting a long swim back.

Always tie yourself to your boat with a fairly long line. An empty canoe or rowing boat can be blown by the wind faster than a man can swim, and if you fall out, your boat may leave you behind. This is especially true of sailing dinghies.

An injured victim

If you are trying to rescue a victim with suspected back or neck injuries, you must be especially careful not to handle him any more roughly than is necessary. The victim should be floated to shore carefully, his body and head being kept as straight as possible. Well-prepared rescuers can often push a flat panel, such as a door or surfboard, under the victim's body and tie him in place with care. Try not to turn his head or bend his back.

Using your clothing to assist you

There are ways you can make your clothing work for you if you are thrown into the water and you believe you'll be forced to keep yourself afloat for a long time. Clothing traps air, and you can take advantage of this.

First, get rid of your shoes. They're dead weight. The close-woven materials which most shirts and jackets are made from will hold air when wet. Not for long, but long enough for you to save your strength between refillings of air in the clothing.

You can tighten your shirt about your neck, perhaps by buttoning the top button. Then blow between the buttons at your chest, underwater if you must, and you'll find that an air bubble forms at the back of the shirt up by your neck. You can also splash air into your shirt by floating on your back, holding up the hem with one hand and ballooning air inside.

You can use your trousers to help you float. You must remove them. Then tie a knot at the bottom of each leg, or tie the legs together. Pull up the zip and blow air into the open top. You then can slip your head between the legs where they have been tied together, holding the waist firmly closed with your hands; or, if they are tied separately, the trousers can serve as water-wings.

If you decide to swim to safety, discarding all your clothes will make the going much easier.

Or you may have to resort to survival floating – simply floating in a natural position, body slumping, head and arms down. When you need air, begin to straighten up. Press your arms downwards and bring your legs together and you'll be lifted enough so that your face will break the surface. Exhale as you lift your face above the water. Then breathe deeply and curl back down to the resting position again. If your body tends to sink, a slight scissors kick can help keep you close to the surface. A gentle finning action with your arms also helps keep you from sinking.

Cramp

There are specific emergencies that can cause a swimmer to panic, unless he has made himself familiar with them and knows what to do.

Cramp always worries swimmers. The muscle tightening of a cramp most frequently affects the hands, feet, arms or legs. Cramp is usually caused by fatigue or over-exertion and is not really dangerous unless you panic. Change your swimming stroke and relax; often the cramp will disappear. If it doesn't, rubbing and kneading the cramped muscle will help. It is important to stretch the muscle. Stretching the muscle and changing your stroke generally relieves the cramp.

Currents

If a swimmer gets caught in a current, he should swim diagonally across the current, even though it may take him out of his way. He will get to safety with less exhaustion.

Undertows and cross-currents tend to drag the swimmer away from the shore. Again, you shouldn't panic or struggle against the current. Instead, swim parallel to shore, across the current and, once you have passed out of its strength, swim to shore.

Remember a simple rule: the sea is much stronger than you are. Don't fight it; yield to it until it releases you.

The unconscious victim

If the person you are trying to rescue is unconscious in the water, get him to shore as fast as you can. Tow him by his shirt collar, his hair or his hand, but keep him on his back and try to keep his mouth and nose up out of the water. If there are other people around, you must, of course, send someone for help and tell others to help you.

An unconscious drowning victim needs help fast, just as the heart-attack victim or choking victim does. If you can't make him breathe on his own in five minutes or so, his body will begin to die. *You must hurry.* You must get air into him in minutes. If his heart has stopped beating, you must give external cardiac compression, just as you would for a heart-attack victim.

If you have reached the victim and he is unconscious and apparently not breathing, you should begin to give mouth-to-mouth artificial respiration as soon as you can, even before you get him all the way out of the water. If you can support his body you should begin breathing into his mouth, using the technique you learned in an earlier chapter.

You remember how:

One, wipe any obvious foreign matter from his mouth.

Two, tilt his head back and lift under the back of his neck.

Three, put the heel of your hand on his forehead to keep it back and, with the fingers of the same hand, pinch his nostrils closed.

Four, blow air into his mouth. Give him a series of quick breaths. Then give him a breath every five seconds in the usual manner.

Start this series right where you are, standing in shallow water, or clinging to the side of the pool, or in a boat, or anywhere you can support the victim on his back and give help effectively. *Speed is vital.*

When you get the victim ashore, lay him on his back, head tilted back in the same way, and continue artificial respiration. If you can't get air into the victim, his throat must be blocked. Look for foreign matter in the back of his mouth. Then recheck to make sure his head is tilted back correctly and that his tongue isn't blocking his throat.

If you feel you must, turn him on his side and give him four sharp blows between the shoulder blades. A child may be suspended momentarily by the ankles or turned upside down over one arm for shoulder-blade blows.

Only after ventilation is established, feel for a pulse in the neck. If you can find none, you must begin external cardiac compression.

Don't bother trying to drain water from his lungs. They won't drain. But if his stomach is bulging, turn him face down for a moment, place both hands under his abdomen and lift him to help empty his stomach. You also can leave him on his back, turn his head to one side and press on his stomach to help drain it.

Do not give up artificial respiration attempts before professional assistance arrives – doctor or police or ambulance – or the victim has been brought to the hospital. From studies of air-breathing aquatic mammals, which can survive oxygen loss for one hour, medicine is discovering more and more about the 'mammalian diving reflex,' in which the body's blood oxygen is reserved for the heart and brain. Humans who have been under water for as much as thirty minutes in water below 70°F have survived.

Recently, an eighteen-year-old student was trapped in a submerged car for thirty-eight minutes. He was pronounced dead, but resuscitation procedures were begun. He regained consciousness after fifteen hours, and two weeks later he returned to college without physical impairment. Seven of nine survivors in a recent study of this subject were children. The diving reflex is even more pronounced in children under three and a half years of age.

If your patient begins to breathe by himself, if his heart is beating by itself and if you're certain he's getting better, don't get overconfident. Even if the victim never was unconscious, neither you nor he should shrug off what has happened.

You should treat the victim for possible shock. This means you must make certain he's breathing easily, elevate his legs and feet about six inches, avoid rough handling, keep him warm and comfortable, keep him lying down and don't give him any food or water. See that a doctor examines him as soon as possible.

Drowning

What to look for

The conscious victim

The unconscious victim

After victim is ashore or aboard a boat

If blockage is suspected in throat

What to do

Treat patient for shock. Make sure breathing is easy.

Lay victim flat on back. Elevate legs and feet. Keep warm and comfortable. Do not give food or water. Get doctor as soon as possible.

Get air into lungs quickly
Begin mouth-to-mouth respiration as soon as possible, even if victim is still in water if it is possible to support body while breathing into mouth.

1. Wipe out victim's mouth.
2. Tilt head back, hand under neck.
3. Heel of hand on forehead, pinch nostrils shut.
4. Blow air into mouth in series of 4 quick breaths. Then 1 breath every 5 seconds.

Lay victim flat on back. Continue artificial respiration.

Turn on side and give 4 sharp blows between shoulder blades.

Administer 4 chest thrusts.

Sweep foreign material from mouth.

Attempt again to ventilate.

After successful ventilation, feel for neck pulse.

If none, start cardiac compression.

If stomach is bulging

Place face down. Put both hands under stomach and lift to help empty.

One can also clear stomach by leaving victim on back and turning head to one side. Press on stomach to clear it.

Continue mouth-to-mouth respiration and cardiac compression until victim revives or help arrives.

Action sequence for drowning victim

1. Lay victim flat on back.

2. Clear mouth of foreign matter.

3. **Commence mouth-to-mouth respiration:**
   - Tilt victim's head back.
   - Place hand under back of neck.
   - Place heel of other hand on forehead and pinch nostrils shut.
   - Blow air into mouth in series of 4 quick breaths, then 1 breath every 5 seconds.

4. If blockage suspected in throat, turn on side and deliver 4 sharp blows with heel of hand between shoulder blades.

5. Administer 4 chest thrusts. Clear foreign material from mouth. Attempt again to ventilate. Repeat blows and thrusts as needed until airway cleared. After successful ventilation, check neck pulse. If no pulse in neck, start cardiac compression.

6. **Continue mouth-to-mouth respiration and cardiac compression until victim revives or help arrives.**

7. You can empty bulging stomach by placing victim on stomach and placing both hands beneath stomach and lifting to help empty it. You can also clear bulging stomach by leaving victim on back, turning head to one side and pressing on stomach to clear it.

8. Protect patient from shock by wrapping in blankets to keep warm. Make victim comfortable and reassure him that everything is all right.

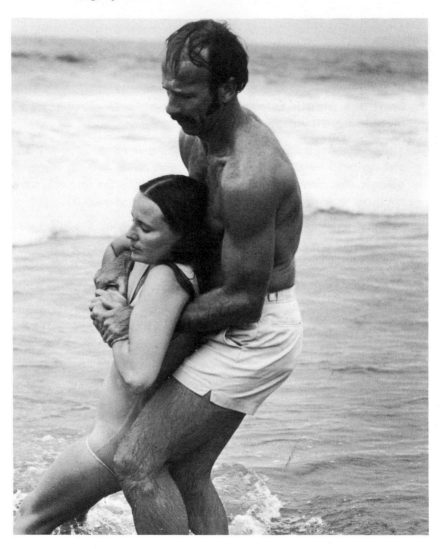

If you see someone in trouble in
the water, you must act fast. Get in
and get them to shore or to the
edge of the pool as quickly as you
can. Be wary of allowing the victim
to get you in trouble.

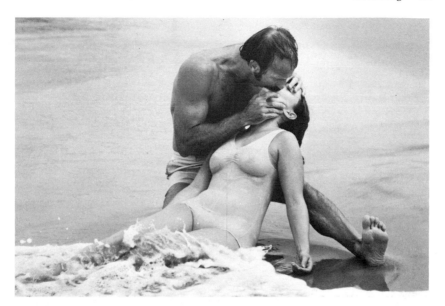

As soon as you are able to stand or get other firm support, such as the side of a pool, deliver four quick, full breaths into the victim's mouth if the victim isn't breathing.

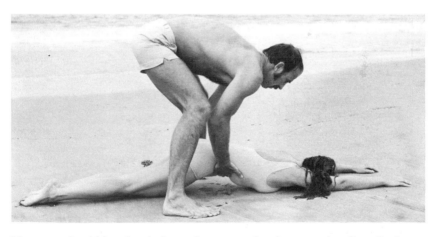

Now you should lay the victim on her stomach, place your hands under her abdomen and lift forcefully. This is called 'breaking' the victim to help force water and air from a bloated stomach.

As soon as you can, call others for help. Volunteers can go for professional assistance or help you with your rescue efforts. Pinch the victim's nostrils and get ready to breathe for the victim.

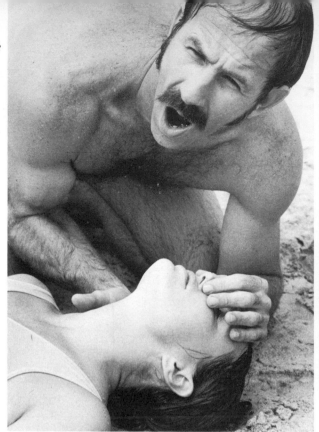

Lift the back of the neck and tilt the head back to facilitate breathing. Pinch the nostrils shut and blow quickly into her mouth. Find out if the airway is clear.

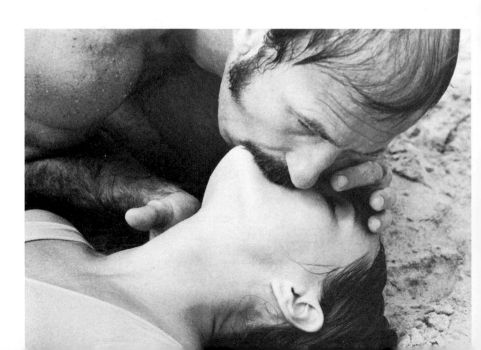

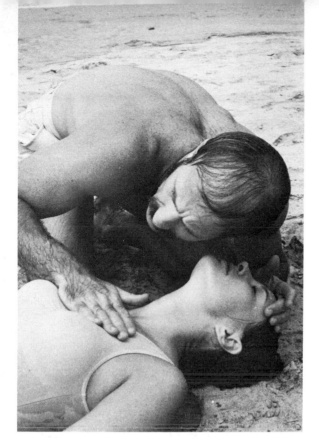

You must find out if the victim is breathing. Look for a rising and falling chest. Feel for movement of the chest. And listen and feel if air is coming from the victim's mouth.

If your attempts to ventilate the victim are unsuccessful, you should roll the victim on her side, moving her carefully as you prepare to deliver blows to the back.

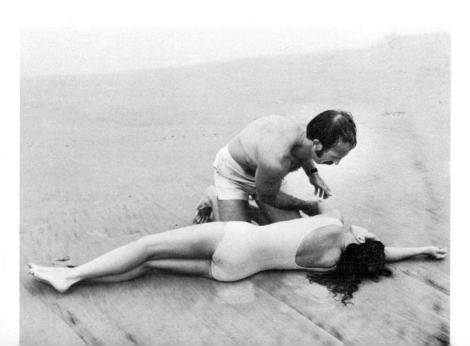

Using the palm of your hand, strike the victim four times between the shoulder blades. Make the blows sharp and firm as you attempt to clear the victim's airway.

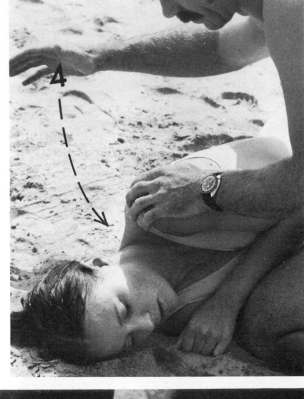

Now roll the victim to her back again. Place your clenched hands between the navel and the lower breastbone and give the victim four abdominal thrusts. This may help clear the airway.

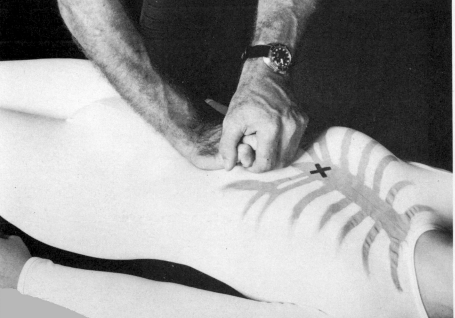

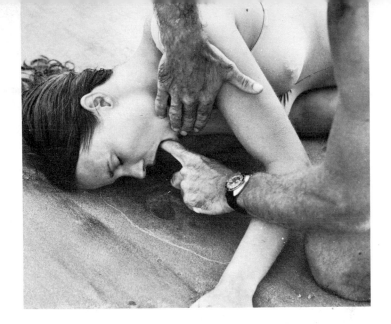

Roll the victim to her side, open the mouth and then probe inside with your finger to see if you have dislodged any foreign body which you may be able to sweep out with your finger.

Roll the victim to her back, open the mouth wide and resume attempts to ventilate. Deliver four quick breaths. Once the victim has air in her lungs, you must check to see if her heart is beating.

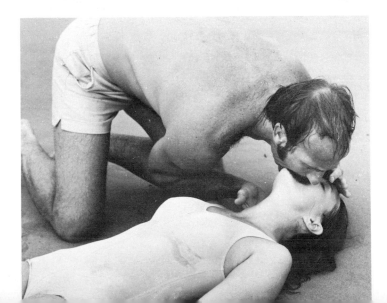

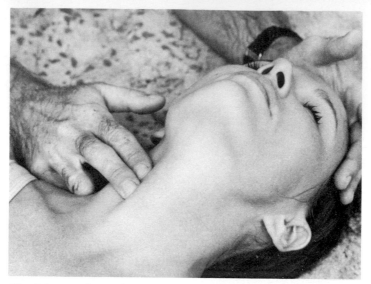

Check for a pulse at the neck, which is the most reliable place to find it. Feel with your fingertips between the windpipe and the large muscle at the front of the neck.

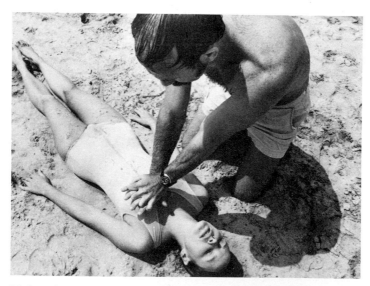

If there is no pulse, locate your hands in the correct place on the lower half of the breastbone, avoiding the cartilage tip. If you are attempting resuscitation alone, give eighty compressions a minute.

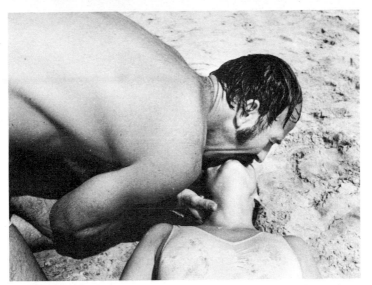

After you have given fifteen compressions, reopen the airway by extending the neck. Once again deliver two quick ventilations without allowing the victim to exhale between them.

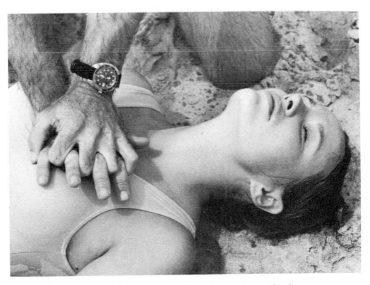

Then you must quickly put your hands back on the lower breastbone and continue the sequence – fifteen compressions alternated with two rapid ventilations.

When help arrives, have the second rescuer ventilate at the rate of one quick breath after every fifth chest compression. Reduce the cardiac compressions to sixty a minute when you are both working.

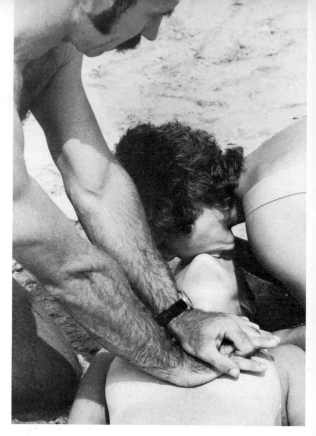

When your patient revives, keep her warm and keep close watch on her breathing and pulse. Get her to professional medical care as fast as you can.

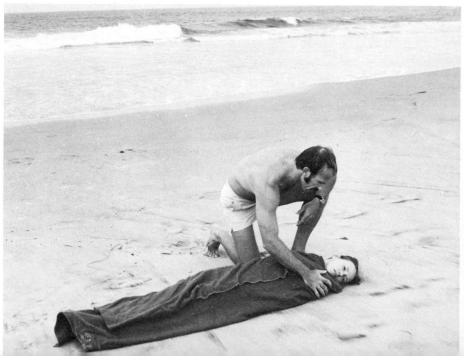

5. Shock

It's time to talk about shock. We have encountered shock already as something to be guarded against in emergency situations and it is all too true – shock is frequently an unwelcome companion to almost all kinds of medical emergencies. Shock can kill.

Shock can take place when, to the untrained eye, there is no reason for it. Shock doesn't really need a reason to happen. It simply happens. It can happen, as we have read, to people rescued from drowning. It can happen to victims of heart attack. Some people go into shock after minor accidents. The sight of blood can send some victims into shock.

The word 'shock' means different things to different people. Shock comes in many different forms and different degrees. All shocks have some effect on the nervous system. But your body responds to small shocks and big shocks in different ways. A woman may faint from the shock she gets when a mouse runs out of a kitchen cupboard. Everyone is familiar with the kind of shock that comes from touching a piece of metal when the body has absorbed static electricity. And, on a more serious level, shock may be caused by a heart attack, an allergic reaction, a serious burn, a spinal injury or loss of blood. All of these affect the nervous system and have a dramatic physical effect on the body.

Let's explore briefly some of the kinds of shock, remembering that you should check victims of every medical emergency for symptoms of shock because shock occurs so often. The danger is always present.

Shock can be caused by loss of blood. If the supply of blood in the body is reduced, this can mean that there is not enough blood to fill the system, and so circulation is cut back. Shock results. Blood volume can be lost in several ways: by external bleeding from open wounds, by internal bleeding from wounds inside the body, and by loss of plasma – the liquid part of the blood – which can happen in cases where the victim is burned or when tissues are crushed.

• Respiratory shock is caused when there isn't enough oxygen in the blood, which happens when the lungs cannot be filled adequately. This can be caused by many things – including chest wounds or broken ribs, obstructions in the throat that cause a victim to choke and damage to the spine that makes muscles paralysed. (We have learned already that the brain needs a great deal of healthy, oxygenated blood.)

• Some shock is caused by loss of control of the nervous system, as when the spine is damaged in an accident. This can result in loss of control of the size of blood vessels. If some blood vessels become widely dilated – too large – they can use up too much of the body's supply of blood. The rest of the body must do without.

• It's true that shock can be caused by fear, bad news, the sight of blood and by minor injuries. Often all these things go together on the battlefield, so that combat soldiers are in danger of plunging into shock when their bodies might otherwise be little affected by wounds. Sometimes minor forms of this kind of shock can result in fainting, and the condition usually corrects itself. If the victim's head is lowered, blood circulates to the brain and normal functions return. A person feeling faint should lower his head at once. Sitting down and dropping the head between the knees usually works.

• Shock can be caused by heart trouble. Proper blood circulation needs an efficient heart, but if the heart doesn't develop the necessary blood pressure to move blood to all parts of the body, circulation is weakened and shock can set in.

• Loss of fluids can cause shock. Therefore a person suffering from dehydration can go into shock. So can someone who has vomited a great deal. Dysentery can cause shock. In all these cases body fluids are being lost, and when that happens shock can result.

So it can be seen that shock is a very real medical emergency. It's not true that shock is a mental thing, a thing always brought on by stress or trauma. It can happen that shock is aggravated by stress, but most shock is a real and physical thing. You can help a victim of shock better if you understand what causes shock. You'll also find it easier to recognize shock if you understand what's happening inside the victim's body.

Stated very briefly, shock is caused by failure to get blood to the tissues of the body and/or not enough oxygen in the blood. In other words, any victim of bleeding or loss of air can fall quickly into shock. If you're going to help save his life, you must be on the look-out for symptoms of shock and you must know what to do about them.

When a victim is in shock, many of his vital body functions are working only marginally. The heart may be feeble. Breathing may be weak. Again, not enough blood is being pumped or not enough oxygen is getting into the blood – or both at once.

Shock can kill as surely as a heart attack, choking, drowning or any other serious medical emergency. Shock can be aggravated by abnormal changes in body temperature, by poor resistance of the victim to stress, by pain, by rough handling and by delay in treatment. So you see that it is necessary that you treat a victim of shock effectively, gently and quickly.

You must always look for shock in any medical emergency. Here's what you should look for:

• The eyes may be dull and without lustre, a sign of poor circulation.

- The pupils of the eyes may be dilated.
- The face may be pale or bluish, which is caused by a lack of oxygen, brought on in this case by reduced circulation.
- Breathing may be shallow, panting, laboured or irregular.
- The pulse may be rapid or weak. This is because the heart is working faster to try to compensate for reduced blood pressure and volume. (You can see what a faithful machine the heart tries to be.)
- The skin may be cold or clammy. This is because the blood has given up effective circulation in the surface areas of the body, especially the hands and feet, and is going to the vital organs.
- There may be nausea, vomiting, anxiety and thirst. The victim may collapse.
- The victim may become apathetic, unresponsive to you or his own condition. He may simply not care. This is because his brain isn't getting enough oxygen. It's slowing down.
- The eyes may eventually become sunken and take on a vacant expression.
- The victim's skin may turn mottled because blood vessels have collapsed. This is a sign that his blood pressure has plunged to a very low level.

Certainly the signs of shock are clear, almost all of them showing up in poor heart and lung action, weakness and bad colour. Now you're going to have to do something about it. You're going to have to move effectively, quickly and gently, or your patient may die.

How to treat shock victims

You know by now that your objectives in helping a shock victim are clear. You must improve circulation of his blood to ensure an adequate supply of oxygen. You must also keep his body temperature constant and as near normal as possible. Often, loss of blood causes shock, so if there is bleeding you must control it at once. And, of course, you should send for professional medical help as soon as you can.

Here are the steps you should take:

First, if your patient is breathing, make certain his throat is clear, then, if unconscious, tilt his head back properly to help keep it open. If he isn't breathing, you must start resuscitation at once.

Second, you must control any bleeding because, as has been pointed out, bleeding can cause shock, and continued bleeding makes it worse. Some bleeding can be controlled by pressure on the wound or by pressure at pressure points (see page 95).

Third, try to make your patient as comfortable as you are able. Ease his pain, if you can. Make him lie down and cover him only enough to prevent loss of body heat. Don't bundle him up so that he becomes too warm. Raising the skin temperature too much is harmful because the heat draws blood back to the skin. This deprives the vital organs of the blood they so desperately need.

The victim's position must be determined by his injuries. If you suspect that his neck or spine is injured, you should not move the victim unless you must to protect him from being hurt even worse.

If your patient is unconscious and has bad wounds of the lower face or jaw, place him on his side to allow fluids to drain away and to help prevent choking on vomit or blood.

A victim who has trouble breathing should be put on his back with his head and shoulders slightly raised. A folded blanket under his head and shoulders will do to lift him about three inches or so.

If you're not sure about the right position for your patient, keep him lying flat on his back. This usually is most restful to his circulatory system. If you have enough blankets, put one under him to help prevent loss of body heat into the ground or other cool surface.

Fourth, a victim in shock may improve if his feet are raised six to twelve inches. This helps to improve blood flow from his feet and legs and may force more blood to his heart and lungs, where a shock victim needs blood badly.

(But be wary. If your patient has head or chest injuries, you must not increase pressure on the injured places. So in these cases do not raise his feet, but instead slightly raise his head and shoulders to ease pressure on the injured areas.)

If your patient becomes less comfortable, if he has more trouble breathing and has new pain after you raise his feet, lower them again.

Remember, whenever you have any doubt about the best position, keep your patient perfectly flat. There won't be any bad effects if you observe this rule, but you may experiment with the other positions if you work gently and carefully. Your patient's general comfort and changes of condition should tell you what positions are best for him.

Fifth, be very gentle with your patient. Avoid rough handling when you can and move him as little as possible, only enough to do your job. Movement may aggravate shock.

Finally, your patient may complain of thirst, and it is true that giving fluids *can* help him fight shock. As we have said, one of the causes of shock is the loss of body fluids – not just blood but all fluids. Dehydration is an ally of shock.

However, in general, you should *not* give your patient anything by mouth – fluids or anything else. Fluids should be given *only* when professional medical help is more than six hours away. Do *not* give your patient anything to eat or drink if he is unconscious, is having convulsions, is vomiting or if you think he is going to vomit. He may force the fluid into his lungs.

Do *not* give fluids to your patient if you think he may need surgery or a general anaesthetic, or if he seems to have a stomach wound. Giving fluids can be harmful if your patient has a brain injury, as additional fluids in the body are likely to cause swelling in the brain, and this is dangerous.

Fluids should be given only if expert help is more than six hours away and if none of the other conditions mentioned is present. Then water may be given at medium temperature, not too hot or too cold. The addition of one teaspoonful of salt and half a teaspoonful of baking soda in each quart of water is beneficial.

Adults may have half a glass of water every fifteen minutes. Children from one to twelve may have a quarter of a glass, and infants an eighth of a glass. If your patient gets nauseated or vomits from the water, don't give him any more.

Remember, a shock victim who can safely take fluids is helped but many victims cannot safely accept fluids, so be careful. **If you're not sure about injuries – including internal bleeding – don't give your patient anything at all by mouth. Never give alcohol.**

Shock is traumatic, so gentle warmth, comfort and easing of pain and stress all help. This means that your personal approach is more important in treating shock victims than in almost any other kind of medical emergency.

So be kind and soothing. Keep your head. You're with your patient to help him. Show him that you know what you're doing – and *that you care* – and he's sure to respond faster. Tender loving care – it's one prescription that always helps your patient.

Shock

What to look for

Dull, lack-lustre eyes. Dilated pupils.

Pale or bluish face. Clammy, cold skin.

Shallow, irregular, laboured breathing. Rapid or weak pulse (throat).

Nausea, vomiting. Thirst, anxiety. Sunken eyes, vacant expression.

Collapse.

If breathing has stopped

If serious bleeding

If head or neck injury

If bad wounds – lower face, jaw

If stomach or chest injury

If dehydration due to thirst, nausea, dysentery, etc.

If extreme fear, loss of control, panic

What to do

1. Place patient flat on back.

2. Make sure throat is clear.

3. Raise head and shoulders.

4. Raise feet 6 to 12 inches (lower if it causes pain).

5. Reassure patient.

Start resuscitation at once.

Control with pressure on wound, pressure points or tourniquet, if necessary. (See pages 94-5.)

Keep body flat.

Place body on side to drain.

On back; no liquids

Small amount of water but only if *no* internal wound or injury and help is more than 6 hours away.

Reassure patient help is coming. Make as comfortable as possible. Calm and soothe.

Action sequence for shock victims

If breathing has stopped, begin resuscitation at once.

1. Ensure adequate breathing:
- Make sure throat is clear.
- Raise feet slightly to improve flow of blood to heart and lungs.

2. Control heavy bleeding:
- Use pressure on wound, pressure points or tourniquet, if necessary (see pages 94-5).
- Elevate the wounded area.

3. Protect injured areas:
- If head or chest injuries, keep body flat on back.
- If face and lower jaw, keep body on side to drain fluids.
- If neck or spine injuries are suspected, **do not move at all**.
- When in doubt, keep victim flat.

4. Give aid and comfort:
- Keep patient warm, but not hot, with blanket or covering.
- Make patient as comfortable as possible. Accede to reasonable requests.
- Be calm and give patient confidence in what you are doing.
- Reassure patient that help is on the way.
- Allay fears. Fear and panic are shock's greatest allies.

6. Poisoning

About 3,000 deaths from poisoning are recorded every year in England and Wales. The majority of poisoning cases are attempted suicides, but about a third are accidents, very often involving substances commonly found in the home.

Medicines, cosmetics, cleaning agents, plant and insect sprays, car fumes, petrol, paraffin, lighter fuel, turpentine, plastic glue, paint, leaves, berries, fungi ... All of these things – and dozens more – are poisonous if swallowed, inhaled, spilled on the skin or injected into the bloodstream.

It is not surprising, since so many dangerous agents are lying around in houses and cars, that children are often the innocent victims of poison. Lack of supervision of children in the home, negligence in storage or disposal of poisonous matter, and curiosity combined with a child's inability to read can lead to tragedy.

The list of dangerous products can go on: aspirin, hair preparations, detergents, dry-cleaning agents, bleach, weedkillers ...

Many of these products have come on the market in recent years, and most of them have no known specific antidote. They can cause breathing to stop suddenly, coma or convulsions, and quick death.

It is obvious that prevention of poisoning is the easiest way of saving a life. Of course, effective treatment is important, and we will tell you what to do; but the first, easiest and most effective thing that you can do is to *keep any poisonous material in your home, garage or farm out of reach of anyone who should not be handling it.*

Common poisonous plants to beware of are foxgloves, laburnums (all parts) and yew (all parts except the red outer part of the berry); deadly nightshade berries; and several species of fungi (including one which is sometimes mistaken for the edible field mushroom).

Alcohol is also a poison. Chronic alcoholism can kill as surely as any other poison. Even in small amounts, alcohol affects physical and mental behaviour and thus endangers the user. Alcohol combined with carbon monoxide often causes motoring accidents. Alcohol and altitude can cause plane accidents. Alcohol and other drugs combined can be deadly. Drink, if you feel you want to, but be careful what you are doing while under the influence and be aware of what other substances you are putting into your body to mix with the alcohol.

There are twenty-four-hour poison information centres in the major cities. Be prepared to give the possible source of the poison and to describe the patient's symptoms. The telephone numbers of the poison centres are as follows:

Belfast	0232 40503
Cardiff	0222 33101
Dublin	Dublin 45588
Edinburgh	031-229 2477
Leeds	0532 32799
London	01-407 7600
Manchester	061-740 2254
Newcastle	0632 25131

The poison centre, or the casualty department of your local hospital, will need to know the victim's age; the name and amount of the poison involved; first aid being given; whether or not the victim has vomited; where you are. You should save the label or container from which the poison came and, if asked, read it to your medical adviser. Often, by examining the contents of a container you can estimate how much has been taken by how much is missing. Finally, save, if you can, a sample of the victim's vomit; medical personnel will probably want to examine it.

Poisons enter the system in four ways, and we will list these ways, tell how each can happen, something about what happens to the body and what you should do to deal with each emergency.

Poisons can harm the body through:
- *Ingestion*, taking poison by mouth
- *Inhalation*, breathing poisonous fumes
- *Absorption*, on and through the skin
- *Injection*, puncturing the skin.

Ingestion, taking poison by mouth

Swallowed poisons may cause nausea, vomiting and diarrhoea. Cramps and severe stomach pain also may be symptoms, and the victim may show slowed breathing and circulation. Often the odour of the poison may be on the victim's breath or there may be stains on his mouth.

Like food, swallowed poison remains in the stomach for a short time before it starts to pass through the intestines. If it can be removed before it leaves the stomach the victim has a better chance of quick recovery. But there are certain cases when the poison should not be removed by vomiting since it might cause further damage.

Do *not* bring on vomiting if the victim has swallowed a strong corrosive poison, one that is *acid* or *alkali*. These poisons include drain cleaner, lye, washing soda, ammonia, bleach and laundry or dishwasher detergent.

These poisons may cause further damage to the throat and oesophagus as they return to the outside. A *petroleum* poison might cause a form of pneumonia if drawn into the lungs through vomiting. If the victim is unconscious or semi-conscious, he might also get vomit into his lungs. If he is convulsing, he should not be made to vomit. If he has a serious heart condition, vomiting may make it worse.

Instead, if he is conscious and not convulsing, give him as soon as possible water or milk to dilute the poison and slow down absorption. Egg white in water may also be used. Two glasses of milk or water are sufficient.

Vomiting *is* called for when the victim has swallowed a non-corrosive poison such as aspirin or snail bait, and poisonous berries or fungi. You can bring it up by giving your patient one tablespoonful of syrup of ipecac, available at the chemist's without a prescription, or you may give him salt dissolved in water to drink. You may tickle the back of his throat, but first dilute the poison with a great deal of water.

Keep his head low to prevent the vomit from getting into his lungs. Remember to collect the vomit so that medical experts can examine it later.

Note: many poisonous substances list the antidotes on the container label. Look for them first. But be careful if it is an old bottle or jar; the antidotes may be wrong. It is best to check with one of the poison centres whose telephone numbers are given above.

Always be alert for signs of shock: shallow breathing, mottled skin, fainting, disorientation.

Inhalation, breathing poisonous fumes

Get your patient into fresh air fast. If he is breathing, get as much fresh air into him as you can immediately. If he isn't breathing, you must give him mouth-to-mouth respiration. If his heart has stopped, you must also administer cardiac compression.

Carbon monoxide is a commonly inhaled poison, and it comes most often from exhaust fumes; sitting in a car with the engine running in an enclosed place is dangerous. Carbon monoxide has no smell and cannot be seen, so often unconsciousness comes with little warning. The victim may feel only a slight headache and dizziness before he is in serious trouble. One symptom of carbon monoxide poisoning is the cherry-red colour of the skin that is unlike any other symptom of illness.

Get your patient into fresh air and help him breathe if he isn't breathing himself; he should be taken to a hospital as soon as possible.

Carbon monoxide and other inhaled poisons cause 900 deaths a year in England and Wales. Motor vehicle exhaust fumes cause about half of these deaths. Other toxic vapours come from petrol, paraffin, lighter fuels, turpentine, plastic glues and paint. Town gas, but not natural gas, is also poisonous.

In all cases, get the victim into fresh air. If you must enter a kitchen, a garage or any enclosed space, use extreme caution. Determine how you are going to get out before you go in. There have been many multiple casualties when the would-be rescuer died with the original victim. Estimate the distance. If you feel that you can make it, take a deep breath, crawl in and hold your breath while dragging the victim out. Be quick. It is best not to try to turn off an engine in a garage filled with carbon monoxide – there may not be time. Concentrate only on your own safety and that of the person trapped. Once out, loosen the subject's clothing and make sure the throat is clear. If the clothing is soaked with a poisonous substance, use gloves to remove it. Then apply plenty of soap and water.

Absorption on and through the skin

Chemicals and corrosives can cause skin burns that need immediate treatment. Some noxious agents can be absorbed through the skin to give rise to systemic effects. Amongst these are the pesticides parathion and malathion, used by farmers; these can cause convulsions after absorption. There are some plants, such as the pot plant, *Primula obconica*, which on contact with the skin cause itching, redness, rash, blisters and occasionally headache and fever; the common nettle causes a lesser but well-known irritating skin reaction.

Treatment consists of removing the victim from the poison and flooding the contaminated skin with water and with soap if available. Unless unconscious or having convulsions, the victim should be given copious fluids to drink. Where medical help is necessary, save the label of the container or provide other evidence of the nature of the poison. Calamine lotion usually copes with nettle stings but medical treatment may be necessary for more severe reactions to plant contact.

Injection, puncturing the skin

Injection of certain drugs and venoms from some insects, spiders and marine animals can cause serious reactions in people sensitive to these substances.

All spiders in Britain are harmless to man; venomous spiders are to be found in most parts of the world, but very few can kill a human being. Scorpions are more dangerous, but are not common in temperate parts of the world. There is only one poisonous snake native to Britain – the adder – and fatalities are extremely rare. (Other snakes which are imported and kept in zoos can of course be poisonous.)

Wasps and bees usually sting only when attacked; if you don't panic and wave your arms about when you see one you are much less likely to be stung.

For minor bites and stings from insects use cold applications – ice wrapped in a towel or cold water. Soothing lotions, such as calamine, also bring relief. Try to remove the sting from the skin by scraping it off with a knife edge or a fingernail, or use some sticky material such as adhesive tape. Avoid squeezing the sting, as this may force more venom into the wound from the poison sacs if they are still attached.

If the reaction is more severe, you should give mouth-to-mouth respiration if it seems necessary. A constricting band (*not* a tourniquet) may be placed a few inches above the injury. Get the victim to a casualty department.

Anaphylactic shock

Anaphylactic shock can occur when the victim is extremely allergic to the substance injected – drugs (including penicillin) or venom from bees, wasps or hornets. Symptoms include itching or burning skin, hives, swelling of the face and tongue, blueness at the lips, a tightening or pain in the chest, wheezing or difficulty in breathing, weak pulse, dizziness, fainting or coma.

Anaphylactic shock requires the injection of medication. Get the patient to expert medical care and remember to pass on information about the substance that caused the reaction. There isn't much else you can do to help.

A sting in the mouth or throat

If someone is stung in the mouth or throat there is a danger that the airway may be blocked by the swelling. Try to control the swelling by giving the victim mouthfuls of cold water, which he should hold in the mouth before swallowing, and place a cold-water compress on the neck. Get the victim to hospital as quickly as possible, but don't let him panic.

Snake bites

There are very few poisonous snakes in Europe, all of them vipers, and a bite from a viper is only very rarely fatal. The common viper, or adder, is the most widespread, and the only one native to Britain. It is distinguished by a dark zigzag stripe down the back. There have been only about ten deaths due to an adder bite in Britain since 1900.

The symptoms may include:

• Shock – the victim feels weak and cold, and may develop a clammy skin and a feeble, rapid pulse.

• Local swelling, which usually develops round the bite within ten minutes. A burning sensation may develop at the site and the swelling may progress up the limb.

• Later symptoms may include vomiting, dizziness, abdominal pain, diarrhoea and even coma.

1. Lay the victim down and reassure him – immobilization delays the spread of the poison.

2. Gently wash the bite to remove any venom around or oozing from the wound. *Do not* cut or suck the wound. If you are far from medical help a constricting band may be applied above the wound, but it must not be too

tight and must be relaxed for one in every fifteen minutes, otherwise gangrene of the limb becomes a real risk.

3. Obtain medical help without delay. *Do not* give alcohol as this can hinder the action of the anti-serum.

Animal and human bites

With animal bites, the problem of infection is made greater – in countries other than Britain – by the possibility of rabies. If the animal has been killed, keep the carcass and pack the head in ice, as it can be examined by a medical laboratory to find out whether the victim should be treated for rabies. (Rabies has been eradicated in Britain by keeping all animals imported into the country in quarantine for six months.)

Finally, human bites can be dangerous because the human mouth is very 'dirty', so there is a considerable danger of infection. Wash the wound with plenty of soap and water.

Poisoning

What to look for	What to do
Ingestion (taken by mouth)	If corrosive poison, *keep down*. If non-corrosive, *bring up*. Send for medical help.
Corrosive: acids or alkalis as in ammonia, bleach, cleaners, detergents, petrol, etc.	**Do not induce vomiting.** Give milk, water, egg white in water.
Non-corrosive: all pills and internal medicines	**Induce vomiting.** Give salt dissolved in water or one tablespoon of ipecac, available at chemists'.
If victim is convulsing	**Do not induce vomiting.**

Antidotes are listed on labels of most poisonous substances. **Poison information services** can be reached by dialling the operator.

Inhalation (breathing in fumes)	Get patient as soon as possible into fresh air, loosen clothing. Send for medical help.
Carbon monoxide or car exhaust fumes may turn skin red. Other toxics include petrol, paraffin, turpentine, glues and paints.	Make sure throat is clear. If poison on skin, wash off with soap and water (hose, shower, sink, bucket).
If not breathing	**Give mouth-to-mouth respiration**
Absorption (on and through skin)	Get victim away from poison. Remove contaminated clothing
Toxic chemicals can burn skin; plants can cause rash and blisters.	Flood skin with large amounts of water and soap for 15 minutes or so.

Injection (puncture of skin)

Stings: venom from stings of insects can be dangerous; anaphylactic shock may occur in person allergic to bees or wasps.

Remove sting by scraping. Use cold application, ice in towel. Place wound lower than heart area. Be prepared to give mouth-to-mouth respiration if necessary. Place constricting band above wound.

Snakebite (puncture or bite): look for puncture marks, local swelling and severe pain; possible convulsions and shock.

Immobilize and reassure victim. Apply constricting band above bite. Wash wound. Obtain medical help.

Action sequence for poisoning cases

If poison container available, check label for antidote.

Phone your local poison information service — see page 77 for telephone numbers.

Swallowed poison	*If a corrosive* (acid, alkali) or petroleum, **do not induce vomiting**. Give patient water or milk. Send for medical help fast.
	If non-corrosive, such as pills, insect powders, any unknown internal medicine, **induce vomiting**. Give patient salt dissolved in water or ipecac to promote vomiting.
Poison inhaled	Get victim to fresh air, away from poison. Remove contaminated clothing.

Poison absorbed through the skin	Get victim away from poison. Flush skin with water and soap. Use hose, shower, sink, even car radiator water.
Poison injected	From insect bites, stings, drugs (including penicillin). Anaphylactic shock may result if person is allergic. If breathing stops give mouth-to-mouth respiration. Use constricting band (a shoelace will do) above wound.
Bites from poisonous snakes	Reduce circulation by using constricting band above the puncture. Keep victim quiet. Wash wound.

7. Drug Overdose

There is some general medical care you can give to a victim of drug overdose. If drugs have been taken by mouth – aspirin and countless other pills are common – induce vomiting as fast as you can. One tablespoonful of syrup of ipecac brings vomiting in fifteen to twenty minutes. So does drinking salt dissolved in water or the finger tickling the back of the throat, if the victim's condition permits it.

If the victim of an overdose is having convulsions, is in a coma or is having trouble breathing, you should make certain that lung and heart action are satisfactory. Use mouth-to-mouth respiration and cardiac compression if they seem called for.

Your patient may become violent. Violence is a symptom of several kinds of drugs. Protect him from hurting himself and others.

And, remember, get your patient to a hospital as fast as you can. Also, if you can, try to identify the drug taken. If there is a suspected container at the scene, send it along with the patient. Experts can identify many drugs by other clues: needle marks on the skin, apparatus such as teaspoons, paper packs, eye droppers, hypodermic needles, vials or collapsible tubes. If your patient can talk, ask him what drug he's taken. Be sure to tell medical personnel what treatment you have given your patient.

Your principal responsibility, if your patient is really ill, is to get him to professional help. That's the best assistance you can give.

There are many kinds of drugs, most of which bring on different kinds of reactions; we'll break them down into their categories and indicate what the dangers are, what symptoms are produced and what you can do to help.

Narcotics

The word 'narcotics' refers, generally, to opium and products derived from opium: paregoric, morphine, codeine. The term also includes drugs derived from morphine: heroin and other substances. There are also laboratory-produced substances that have morphine-like effects on the body: meperidine and methadone.

Even with a normal dose of narcotics, a patient can have some unpleasant side-effects, including sweating, nausea, vomiting, dizziness and constipation.

Narcotics can cause lethargy, sleep and often coma when taken in overdose. Other effects include depression of breathing (including eventual respiratory failure), sweating, lowered temperature in the body, relaxed muscles and contraction of pupils to pinpoint size. In short, narcotics depress. They slow down the body so that mind and muscle go slack.

Most of these drugs are habit-forming, and the victim can come to depend on them. A 'hooked' victim who needs a larger dosage shows nervousness, restlessness and anxiety. He may cry and his nose may run. He may have hot and cold flushes. He may yawn a great deal and get aches in his muscles. His appetite and weight will go down. His pupils will become large when he is 'between fixes'. He will experience increased respiration rate, blood pressure and body temperature. He will, of course, have an intense craving for a 'fix'.

Treatment. Keep the victim awake. Keep him breathing and be prepared to do mouth-to-mouth respiration. This may be all that is necessary to keep the severely overdosed patient alive. Make certain, if he has vomited, that he isn't choking on it. Keep him at an even temperature with necessary clothing and blankets. Get medical help at once.

Hallucinogens

Hallucinogens are what they sound like: drugs that can produce hallucinatory mood changes, often of a bizarre nature. There can be disturbances of self-awareness, sensations, thoughts and emotions. Time and depth perception can be altered, and there can be both illusions and delusions.

Drugs that can bring on these sensations are lysergic acid diethylamide (LSD), mescaline and several other synthetic drugs. These drugs have no accepted medical use.

They are usually taken irregularly, but often they are taken several times a week. Users may want to repeat because of psychological but not physical need.

They can cause nervousness, a faster heartbeat, higher blood pressure, higher body temperature, enlarged pupils and a flushed face. The psychological effects cannot be predicted – they can be up or down.

Such drugs can also cause loss of emotional control, delusions, hallucinations, depression, tension and anxiety.

Treatment. Protect your patient from harming himself and try to talk him down in a safe and peaceful place. Get him to a doctor fast. It's better if two people go with him.

Stimulants

Stimulants, or uppers, increase a user's thought rate and they offset sleepiness and fatigue.

Among them are bennies, pep pills, Dexedrine, speed, crystal and others. They come in many names, colours and shapes. Caffeine and cocaine are also stimulants. Coffee now and then won't hurt you, but large doses of caffeine can be dangerous. Cocaine is a powerful stimulant to the nervous system.

The effects are plain enough: wakefulness, alertness, relief from fatigue, a feeling of well-being. These drugs can reduce craving for food and often have been used for this purpose.

Abuse of these drugs can cause dependence in the mind, but not the body, so that withdrawal can be accomplished without serious trouble as a rule. The body can learn to tolerate large amounts of the drugs so that dosages must be increased for effect.

Abuse can cause confusion, disorganization, irritability, suspiciousness, fear and compulsive repetition of small, meaningless acts. After a 'run', the user is drained, weepy, depressed and terribly hungry.

Treatment. Protect your patient from himself, make sure he is breathing normally, keep his body temperature normal and get him to psychiatric help.

Sedatives, tranquillizers and hypnotics

Amongst these are the barbiturates (e.g. sodium amytal and nembutal) also Doriden, Miltown (meprobamate), Librium (chlordiazepoxide), Valium (diazepa), chloral and paraldehyde.

Overdosage with these drugs causes drowsiness and then a deepening unconsciousness, lowering of body temperature and blood pressure, and the danger of eventual respiratory failure. Alcohol can potentiate the depressant effect of these drugs, substantially reducing the minimal lethal dosage.

If confronted with a patient still conscious despite overdose with this group of drugs, induce vomiting and obtain medical help; if already unconscious, maintain respiration until medical help is obtained.

Inhalants

Inhalants are the latest attraction for far too many young people. Inhalants include fast-drying glue or cement, many paints, lacquers, thinners, removers, petrol, paraffin, lighter fuel, dry-cleaning fluid, nail polish and nail-polish remover.

Often the user will soak a cloth with the substance and hold it over his nose and mouth. Or he may put a paper or plastic bag with the substance in it over his head to get the fumes into his body. It is dangerous in any case to place a plastic bag over the head, as suffocation can result.

The user gets a sort of drunken sensation, feeling dizzy and somewhat high. Eventually it can lead to depression that can even result in unconsciousness.

Some of the propellants in aerosols are poisonous to the heart and can cause death by changing the rhythm of the heartbeat. The liver and other organs can be affected as the user's dependence on the drugs grows.

Treatment. Get the patient to fresh air, removing the source of inhaled poison. If his breathing falters, give him artificial respiration. Get medical help.

Alcohol

Yes, alcohol is a dangerous drug, too. Too much drinking can cause social and financial ruin and cause physical damage to the body. Alcohol taken with a barbiturate or a tranquillizer can be very dangerous.

The excessive drinker needs your help. If he has drunk to the point of passing out, help him sleep it off quietly. If he shows signs of shock (clammy skin, weak and rapid pulse, abnormal breathing), he needs medical help. Keep him warm, make certain he is breathing well enough and if he vomits, don't let him choke.

Later, when he is better, encourage him to seek help from Alcoholics Anonymous.

Drug Overdose

What to look for

If there is lethargy, sleep, coma, shallow breathing, sweating, contraction of pupils to pinpoint size, user has been on **narcotics** (opium, morphine, codeine, heroin, meperidine, etc.).

If there is loss of emotional control, delusions, hallucinations, depressions, tension, anxiety, user has been on **hallucinogens** (LSD – lysergic acid diethylamide, mescaline, psilocybin).

If there is confusion, disorganization, irritability, suspiciousness, fear, repetition of small, meaningless acts, if drained, weepy, terribly hungry, user has been on **stimulants** (Dexedrine, Methedrine, pep pills, etc.).

If drug effect is unconsciousness, lower body temperature and danger of respiratory failure, user has been on **tranquillizers or sedatives** (Miltown, Equanil, Librium, Valium, barbiturates, etc.).

What to do

Keep patient awake. Get medical help at once. If breathing slows or is shallow, begin mouth-to-mouth breathing.

Protect patient from harming himself. Get to doctor fast. Best if two people escort patient to doctor for better control of patient. Reassure.

Protect patient from self and get to psychiatric help quickly.

Keep patient awake if possible. Maintain airway. Get to doctor fast.

If there is a drunken feeling, dizziness and a high leading to a depression, user has been on **inhalants** (fast-drying glue, paints, thinners, removers, etc.).

If patient's breath falters, give artificial respiration. Get medical help.

Remember, in all these cases, if breathing stops, mouth-to-mouth respiration can save a life.

User has been taking **alcohol**; he may show signs of shock.

Allow victim to sleep it off. If in shock, get medical help. Make sure he does not choke.

Action sequence for drug overdose

Narcotics Heroin, morphine, dope, junk, hard stuff, H, horse, etc.	Keep patient awake. Get medical help at once. Do mouth-to-mouth respiration if his breathing slows or stops.
Hallucinogens LSD, cubes, Big D.	Protect patient from harming self. Get to medical help quickly. Better if two persons escort patient to help for control purposes.
Stimulants Dexedrine, cocaine, speed, dexies, bennies, uppers, etc.	Keep patient from harming self. Get to psychiatric help.
Sedatives, tranquillizers and hypnotics Valium, Librium, barbiturates, etc.	Keep patient awake and moving if possible. Maintain airway in unconscious patient. Get medical help fast.

Volatile chemicals
Glue, petrol, paraffin, lighter and cleaning fluids, nail polish and remover, quick-drying paints and thinners, etc.

If patient's breath falters, give artificial respiration. Get medical help.

Alcohol
Wine, beer, spirits, etc.

Patient will usually sleep it off. However, he may choke on his own vomit or partly regurgitated matter stuck in the throat. Prevent choking, using methods on pages 38 ff. Watch out for shock.

8. Accident Injuries

Guess what the leading cause of death is among people one year old to thirty-eight years old. That's right, accidents – and accidents remain one of the most frequent causes of death throughout our lifetime.

Just imagine the total annual cost of medical attention, the loss of earnings, property damage and insurance costs because of accidents. It comes to millions of pounds, even if you don't include the toll in pain, suffering, disability and personal tragedy, which cannot be costed.

If you know what to do for an accident victim, and if you act promptly and with common sense, you can reduce much of the cost and suffering and heartbreak that so often accompany accidents. And if you can give proper first aid, this is an even greater service, because accidents happen in strange places, often where medical aid is not available.

Another advantage of proper first aid knowledge and practice is one that we have encountered earlier: if you know how to help others, you are often better able to care for yourself should you become a victim. If you are injured in such a way that you cannot help save your own life directly, you might be able to tell other rescuers what to do.

There is no finer satisfaction than that which comes from relieving suffering and saving life; but there is another side to the coin; well-meaning attempts to help can do more harm than good if not backed up by a basic knowledge of first aid.

George is hurt when he falls down a flight of stone steps. His leg is broken. It's a simple fracture and there doesn't seem to be anything else wrong with George. When the well-meaning spectators reach George they help him to his feet. He can't stand, and his broken leg gives way. The broken ends of bone slide past each other and grate into more bone and soft tissue.

George falls again and now his 'rescuers' pick him up and carry him to the kerb, his broken leg dangling. Blood vessels and muscles are torn and the sharp ends of the broken bone comes through the skin to the outside, resulting in a lot of bleeding and a frightening scene of disaster in the red mess that follows.

George is placed on the pavement and a coat is put under his head to prop it up. Somebody straightens his crooked leg, shoving the bones back inside the now jagged wound. Going inside with the bone are bits of dirt, trouser cloth and God knows what else.

The ambulance arrives and George is rushed to the hospital. In the emergency room the doctors shake their heads, wondering what sort of accident has mangled their poor patient so badly.

It's important that you should learn what *not* to do, as well as what you *ought* to do.

Here are a few basic and simple rules that apply to almost any treatment of an accident victim, including accidents that range from broken limbs and bullet wounds to simple bumps and bruises.

1. Don't move the victim, except to get him away from danger, until you are certain that movement will not worsen his injuries.

2. Make certain your patient is breathing. If he isn't, check to be sure his airway is clear and then give mouth-to-mouth or mouth-to-nose artificial respiration. It's useless to tend the wounds of a patient who is dying because he is unable to breathe. Check for pulse in the neck. If patient is unconscious and has no pulse, begin resuscitation.

3. Control severe bleeding. If a victim loses a quart of blood (a pint for children) or more, he'll easily slip into shock because there isn't enough blood to feed the vital parts of his body.

Remember these three steps. No matter what else you must do to help an injured victim, you've got to take care of these things first. Once your victim is in a safe place, once you know he's breathing and once you've controlled heavy bleeding, then you can begin to treat his wounds. You'll have more time to plan, to think and to do a better job because you'll have treated his vital life-support needs first.

Now you can examine your patient with care. Examine him for open wounds and discolorations which might indicate there is something wrong inside. Loosen his clothing if you think it will make him more comfortable, but don't tug at his belt. You could make a spinal injury worse. Examine him for shock. Try to be gentle and soothing.

Check your patient's pulse, his eyes, the size of his pupils. Look for paralysis, examine the colour of his skin. In short, look for all the symptoms indicated earlier. They'll help you determine how seriously your patient is hurt and help you decide what you must do.

Check to see who your patient is, if you think it's necessary. If he is unconscious, you may need to dig out a wallet to help identify him and to have relatives notified. It's a good idea to have witnesses when you are searching a victim.

If you seem to be the most capable rescuer present, you must remain on the scene, doing what you can to help until professional aid arrives.

Wounds

We've all seen lots of wounds. When a child scrapes his knee, when you get a black eye by running into a door, when you bruise yourself on the elbow, when you cut your finger with a kitchen knife. These are wounds, internal and external.

An external wound is one that breaks the skin. Here the dangers can be immediate and serious: infection and excessive bleeding. Cuts or lacerations (jagged cuts) can bleed a great deal, while a puncture wound may bleed very little. The bleeding from an open wound reduces the danger of infection, while a puncture, although it looks neat and harmless, often is much more dangerous because the wound has not flushed itself by bleeding and because a foreign (and dirty) object has been thrust into the body.

Any wound from which blood escapes, which persists in bleeding even though you have tried to stop it, which is a deep puncture, which leaves a foreign object in the body, which comes from an animal or human bite, or which seems to have severed or crushed nerves, tendons or muscles should be seen by a doctor as fast as possible.

How to control bleeding

Even severe bleeding can usually be stopped or slowed satisfactorily by direct pressure of your hand over the wound. You should use a pad of clean cloth. Sterile gauze is ideal, but any soft clean cloth can do the job. In the absence of cloth, your bare hand or fingers may be used, but you must try to keep the wound as clean as you can.

If blood soaks into the cloth, don't remove the cloth. Leave the wound undisturbed and add more cloth on top, then press more firmly with your hand.

By applying pressure in this way you are seeking to stop the bleeding without stopping normal blood circulation underneath. In other words, it is always safer to apply uniform pressure along the contours of the body than to thrust sharply into the soft parts of the body. This latter can interrupt the flow of blood, with serious consequences.

When the bleeding seems to be slowing satisfactorily, tie the bandage in place, firmly enough to remain snugly over the wound but not so tight that it cuts off circulation. If redness develops around the wound, if your patient complains of pain or if he tells you that the area around the injury feels numb, you must loosen the bandage. It's cutting off his blood flow, and this can cause more harm than the wound itself.

The wounded area should be raised above the level of your patient's heart; this reduces blood pressure and, thus, the bleeding.

If direct pressure and elevation don't stop the bleeding, you should put finger pressure on the artery that is supplying blood to the wound. In doing this, you are compressing the artery against the bone underneath, squeezing it closed to cut off or slow the flow of blood to the wound. This also stops the flow of blood between the pressure point and the extremity of the body, so that it is dangerous and should be used only when there is no other way to stop the bleeding.

To relieve a severely bleeding arm wound, apply pressure over the artery about midway between the armpit and the elbow, with the flat surface of your fingers doing the pressing as you grip the arm. The pressure point is on the inside of the arm, in the groove between the large muscles.

To relieve bleeding from an open leg wound, press your hand against the femoral artery. The pressure point is on the front of the thigh, just below the middle of the crease of the groin where the artery crosses over the thigh bone on its way to the leg. When you do this, place your patient on his back and press with the heel of your hand.

Use of these arm and leg pressure points should be accompanied by the same efforts to control bleeding that you made earlier with direct pressure on the wound and by elevating the wound above the heart.

Beware of tourniquets. A tourniquet is very efficient for stopping the flow of blood – usually all too efficient. A tourniquet should not be used except in a critical emergency after direct pressure on the correct pressure point has failed to stop severe bleeding. In other words, your patient should be in danger of bleeding to death before you resort to a tourniquet.

When a tourniquet is properly applied, it stops the flow of blood completely beyond the point of application. If it is left in place for too long, tissues will die from lack of blood and oxygen. Usually when a tourniquet is removed or loosened, the bleeding resumes with a rush because of the build-up of blood pressure.

If you decide to use a tourniquet, it means *you're choosing to risk the loss of a limb* in order to save your patient's life.

If you've made such a decision, place the tourniquet just above the wound, wrapping a band of cloth, a belt or other *flat* material (not wire, string or rope, which cut into tissue), rolled into a thin strip, around the limb. Tie a knot, place a stick or other firm and straight object over the knot and tie it on with another knot. Now you should be able to twist the stick and so tighten the tourniquet until the bleeding stops. Then tie the stick in place to keep it tight enough to keep the bleeding stopped.

If your patient's limb has been torn off in an accident, you need have no hesitation about using a tourniquet just above the stump. The limb is lost, and doubtless your action is helping to save the victim's life.

Write a note about the location of the tourniquet and the time it was applied, and attach the note to your patient's clothing where it can easily be seen. Treat the victim for shock and give any other first aid necessary. *Never cover a tourniquet.* Keep it in sight where other rescuers can easily spot it.

Prevention of infection

If you have stopped a bleeding wound with a compress, don't remove the pad in order to clean the wound. You'll probably make the bleeding start again, and that's a worse danger than infection.

However, if the wound has not bled severely and if the tissues are not cut deeper than the skin, the wound should be cleansed thoroughly before it is dressed and bandaged.

To cleanse a wound, wash your hands with soap and water and then wash the wound with ordinary toilet soap or a mild detergent. Flush the wound with plenty of fresh water. Then *blot* the wound dry with a sterile pad and apply a clean dressing and bandage.

Don't dig into a deep wound to remove foreign objects. You're liable to make the wound more severe and increase the danger of infection. However, you may remove nails, fishhooks (push them through and snip off the barbed end, then bring the shaft back out of the original entry hole) and other objects which don't seem to be deep or penetrating vital areas. Don't try to move an impaled victim, unless you must to save his life. And don't probe for a bullet inside the body, no matter what you've seen in television westerns.

An infected wound shows these signs: swelling, redness, a sensation of heat, throbbing pain, tenderness, fever, pus (beneath the skin or draining) and red streaks leading from the wound, which indicate that infection is spreading.

To treat infection, you should keep the infected area immobilized and your patient lying down, preferably in bed. Reduction of physical activity helps slow the spread of infection.

Elevate the infected area, if you can. Apply heat to the infection with hot water bottles, or warm, moist towels. Towels wrapped in plastic, foil or waxed paper retain their heat longer. Keep applying heat until you get your patient to a doctor.

Above all, get your patient to professional medical help; any delay could be dangerous.

Closed wounds

A simple black eye is a closed wound, but so are much more dangerous injuries: broken bones, massive damage to soft tissues such as muscles, blood vessels and nerves, and damage to vital organs.

Look for pain and tenderness to determine if there is a closed wound in your patient. Also look for discoloration, uncontrolled restlessness, excessive thirst, vomiting or coughing up of blood or passage of blood in the body wastes. Also watch for shock – cold, clammy skin, very rapid but weak pulse, rapid breathing, dizziness or unconsciousness.

Keep your patient quiet and unmoving, if possible. You cannot determine the extent of his internal injuries. Keep him breathing and don't give him anything to drink if you think he is damaged inside.

Minor wounds (that black eye again) call for cold applications to reduce swelling and slow down internal bleeding. Save your beef-steak for a celebration dinner after your patient is well.

Fractures

A fracture is a break or a crack in a bone. A closed or simple fracture means that the broken bone didn't come through the skin to the outside. An open or compound fracture is one in which broken ends of the bone protrude from the body. Open fractures are much more serious because of the danger of infection.

Most broken bones are caused by motor vehicle accidents, falls and violent sports. Often older people can break their brittle bones very easily.

Usually a conscious victim can tell you if any of his bones are broken. The pain can be severe, he may report a grating sensation on bone ends, he may have heard a bone snap or he may have trouble moving a broken limb.

Other signs of broken bones are: obvious deformities and differences in shape and length of bones on either side of the victim's body, swelling, pain or tenderness when you press against a suspected fracture. Only a doctor can make an accurate diagnosis, but when any of these signs are present you should suspect broken bones. Even if the injury is only a sprain, it's wise to treat it as a fracture. Movement and rough handling are never good for a patient.

First aid for broken bones

There are several important steps you must take at once.
1. Make sure your patient is breathing.
2. Stop any heavy bleeding.
3. Treat your patient for shock, if necessary.
4. Don't handle him roughly. If possible, he should not be moved at all. Remember, it's easy to damage further a fracture wound by moving the victim.

You must send for medical help, of course. But if none is available quickly you might have to move the victim from the scene of the accident. In this case, you must immobilize the fracture area first. You should *not* attempt to set (reduce) a fracture, even though you've seen them do it a thousand times in the movies. You may well aggravate the wound and leave your patient in a worse condition than before.

If your patient has an open fracture, you should treat the exposed wound. Cut away clothing over the wound and apply pressure with a sterile pad to slow bleeding. Do not wash the wound, do not probe into it, do not stick your fingers inside the wound. The danger of infection is extremely high.

If a piece of bone is protruding, try to cover the entire wound with clean compress pads, or clean sheets or towels. Do not replace the bone fragment – it may already be contaminated.

Treat open fractures before you treat closed fractures, and keep the affected limb elevated, if you can.

Neck fractures should be suspected in any accident victim with serious head injury or with neck pain – especially if it radiates down the arms. Tingling or paralysis of the arms or legs is especially serious. The neck should be splinted by wrapping a wide folded towel or folded newspaper around the neck to prevent movement and should be held absolutely still the whole time by a rescuer. Do not bend the neck forward or to the side, and avoid any rotation.

Splinting

If you must move your patient, you'll probably need to splint the area of the break. The purpose, of course, is to keep the limb immobile so that the broken bone ends do not grate or tear tissues. Many simple fractures have been turned into compound fractures because of careless handling.

It's not likely that you'll have commercial splints handy when you need them, so you must improvise. An injured leg can be secured snugly against the uninjured one, with padding between, if possible. An injured arm may be padded and bound snugly to your patient's chest or to his side, depending on whether his arm is straight or bent.

A pillow will serve as a splint if it can be tied or pinned around a fracture. Corrugated cardboard makes good splints when it is bent along the creases to form a three-sided box to cradle arms or legs. The splints should be long enough to pass the joints on either side of a fracture and they ought to be padded before being tied snugly with string, rope or strips of cloth every few inches. You can also tie splints into place with neckties, belts or any other strong material that can be made to stay in place.

Be wary. If your patient complains of numbness, tingling or an inability to move his fingers or toes, loosen the splint ties. They probably are dangerously tight and cutting off the flow of blood.

Keep checking your patient for shock, breathing, heartbeat and general comfort. Treat him gently and be reassuring until professional help arrives.

Accident Injuries

What to look for	What to do
The first steps	Don't move patient unless in a dangerous area. Send for medical help immediately.
1. Check breathing.	If patient not breathing, clear throat. Give mouth-to-mouth respiration.
2. Check for bleeding.	Look for wounds and bleeding. Control severe bleeding.
Examine for shock. Check pulse, pupils of eyes and colour of skin.	Keep warm. Make comfortable. Reassure that help is on way.
Open wounds, severe bleeding	Apply pressure on wound in form of cloth, pad or compress. Keep compress applied. Add new cloths on top of compress if necessary.
	Use pressure points, strips of cloth, etc. Use a tourniquet only to save the patient from bleeding to death.
Closed wounds, internal injury Pain and tenderness, swelling and discoloration, broken bones and damage to internal organs. Restlessness and thirst, vomiting and coughing up blood. Shock.	Keep patient quiet and unmoving if possible. Keep him breathing and do not give anything to drink if internal injury suspected.

Fractures – simple (skin unbroken)

Conscious patient will help find fracture. Look for obvious deformities in shape and size of bones, swelling, tenderness, pain.

Immobilize limb.

Keep patient quiet and calm. Don't allow patient to move.

Fractures – compound (skin broken)

Treat open wound; cut away clothing over wound and apply pressure to halt bleeding. Do not wash or probe wound. Do not attempt to put bone back. Cover wound and fracture with cloth.

Splinting

If patient must be moved, splint the fracture.

Secure injured leg against whole one. Fractured arm can be secured to body to immobilize.

Action sequence for accident injuries

1. Do not move patient unless you must. Send for medical help.

2. Make sure patient is breathing and heart is beating.

3. Control heavy bleeding with compression on wound, or with pressure points; in a matter of life and death a tourniquet may be used.

Check body for injuries and signs of shock. Give comfort and aid. Send some persons for help and use others to help you with patient.

Fractures
- Do not move the patient, unless in dangerous area.
- Keep compound fracture area clean. Stop bleeding and be wary of shock. Do not try to set the bone. Cover fracture wound after checking the bleeding.
- Splint broken bones if you have to move the patient.
- Extend splints past limb joints.
- Do not splint so tightly that the circulation is cut off.

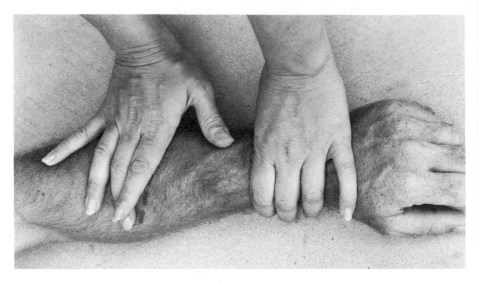

You might ease the flow of blood by applying pressure with your fingers on both sides of the wound. This would give you or your helper more time to prepare bandages or to get help.

The safest way to control bleeding is to apply direct pressure over the wound. Use a clean dressing, preferably something sterile. Press it evenly and as firmly as necessary on the wound.

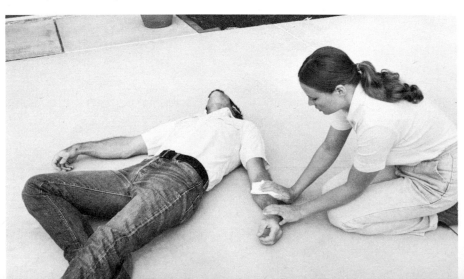

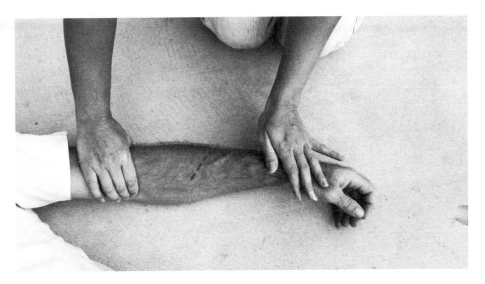

If direct pressure doesn't stop the flow of blood, you may apply pressure on the so-called pressure points, which are located where a large artery passes over a bony prominence.

Finally, tie a bandage in place over the wound. Start by placing clean cloth directly over the wound, after you have treated the open wound as best you can.

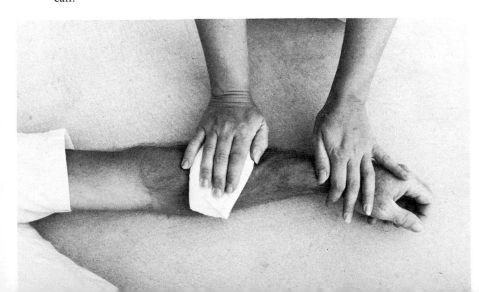

Secure the bandage in place by tying it loosely enough to permit circulation, yet tightly enough to make sure that it stays where you want it and that it keeps the wound clean and prevents bleeding. Get help.

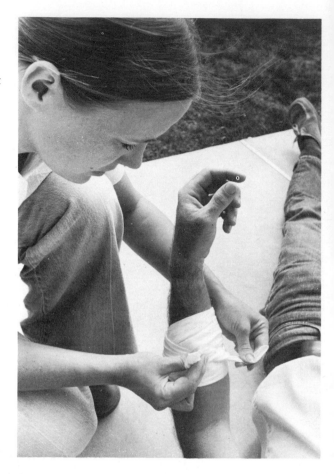

A folded newspaper or a magazine serves well as a splint when you are treating a fracture of the forearm. Move the arm very carefully to prevent further damage to your patient.

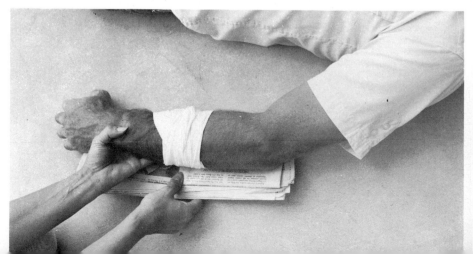

Strips of cloth torn from the victim's shirt make adequate ties for binding the splint in place. Again, rough treatment of the victim will cause further injury.

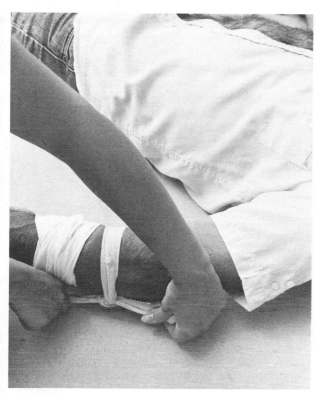

Continue tying strips of cloth. Idcally, you should immobilize the joint below and the joint above the fracture. The idea is to keep the injured bone as secure as possible.

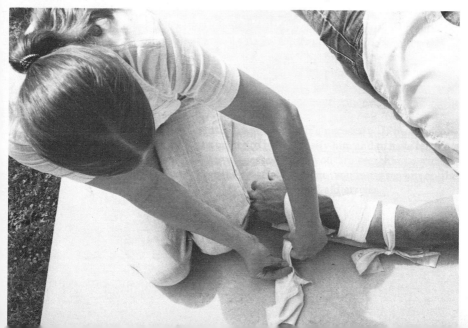

This is how the splint should look when you have secured it correctly. Note that the victim's arm was placed on a flat surface for support while the treatment was being performed.

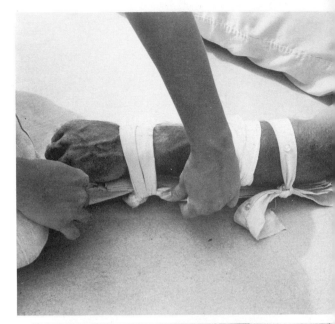

Here the rescuer is checking the pulse below the splint to make certain the ties have not dangerously slowed the flow of blood.

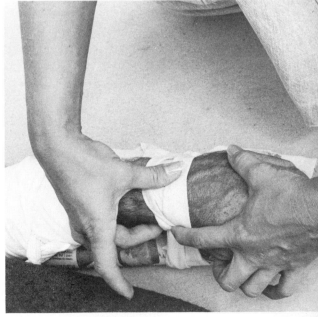

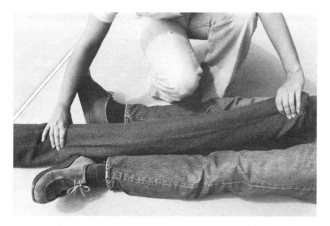

If necessary, you may place a folded blanket between the victims legs. This will help pad the limbs to keep them from being further damaged. Any soft padding material should help.

Now you have the pad between the victim's legs as you get ready to bind the victim's legs together to allow the good leg to be a splint for the damaged leg. Handle your patient gently.

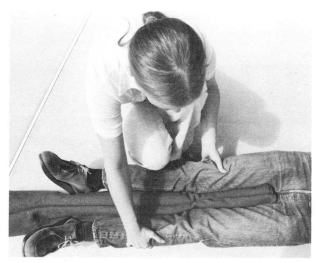

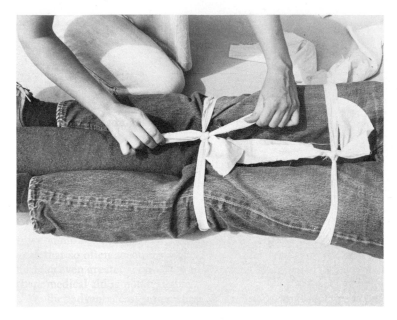

Here the rescuer is using strips of cloth from the victim's shirt to secure the legs, so that the good leg will immobilize the injured leg. Handle the patient carefully to avoid further damage.

Here is the finished treatment. Note that the padding is evenly in place, that the legs are tied firmly in several places, tightly enough to immobilize the legs but not enough to injure them.

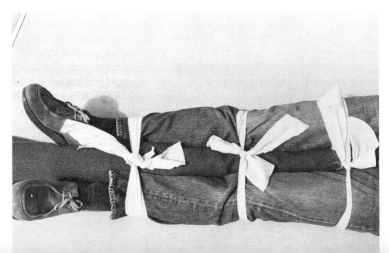

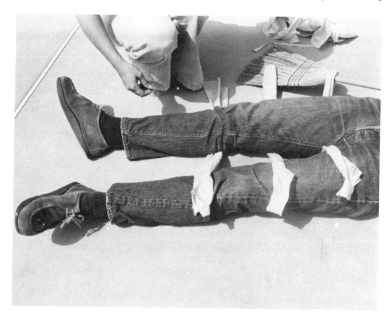

Prepare to splint a fracture of the leg by first placing the ties beneath the victim's leg. Be very careful not to move the injured part of the body any more than is necessary.

Here we have the ties all in place, prepared for application of the splint. Do not attempt to set a displaced broken bone yourself. Usually you will only make the victim's condition worse.

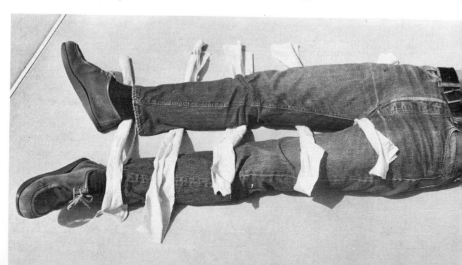

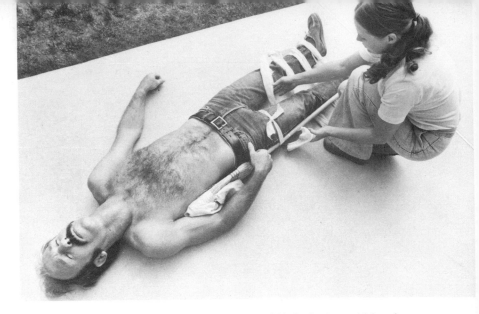

You may use a broom as an improvised splint, if it is the best aid handy. Secure it with the ties you have already placed under the victim's leg, working gently all the time.

Be sure to tie the splint ties the entire length of the splint, using as many ties as you can. The more ties, the more secure will be the injured limb. The broken bone must not move.

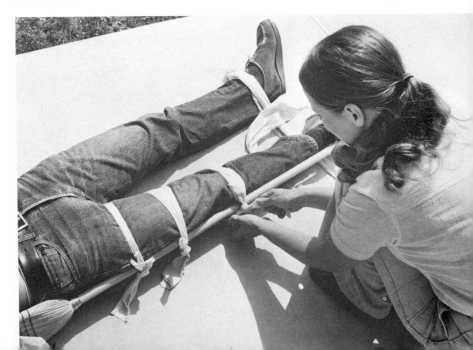

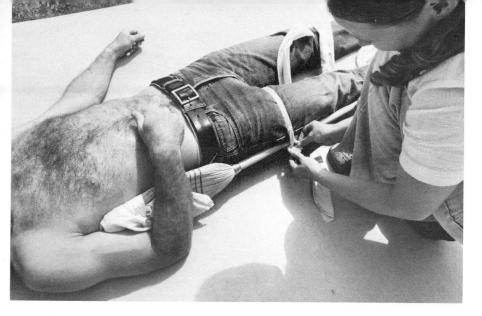

You can prevent the straws of the broom splint from injuring the victim's underarm by tying a piece of cloth over the bristles, thus padding them and making the patient more comfortable.

Check the knots you make in the splint ties to make sure that they are firm enough not to come loose when the victim is moved by rescuers. Note that the knots are placed so that they can be untied without moving the victim.

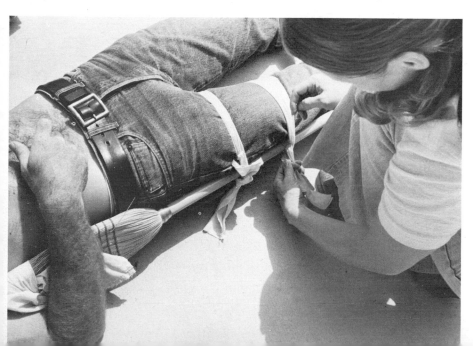

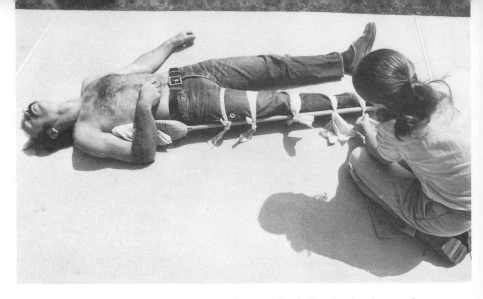

Now you have the splint completely in place, with all ties also in place and knotted properly. Be sure to keep the victim lying flat, unmoving and as comfortable as you can make him.

Here's a close look at the area where the foot pulse is located. If the splint ties are so tight that they have impeded blood circulation, loosen them at once and re-tie them more safely.

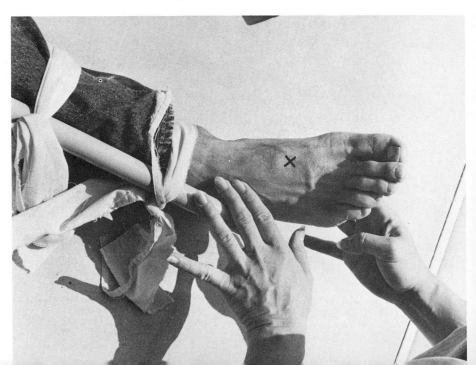

9. Fire and Burns

Burns can be among the most painful, agonizing, disfiguring, time-consuming and expensive to treat of all injuries. A thousand people in England and Wales lose their lives from burns or smoke each year. Most of these are under fourteen or over sixty-four years old.

We've all heard about the causes of fires and the tragic burns that result: carelessness with matches and cigarettes; scalds from hot liquids in the kitchen; defective cooking, heating and electrical equipment; open fires that get out of hand; certain chemicals such as lye, acids and detergents – and even the sun itself.

These horrifying casualties could be greatly reduced if we all took more care, observed simple precautions and knew what to do in the event of fire.

Precautions in the home

Solid fuel fires. Do not use inflammable liquids to assist lighting. Always use a fireguard with a fine mesh and attach it securely. Do not place mirrors over the fireplace. Have your chimney swept regularly.

Other heaters (oil, electric, gas, etc.). Do not drape clothes over the guard. Have all heaters serviced regularly, especially oil heaters, and use a fireguard even if the appliance has an integral guard.

Cooker. Have it well away from curtains, cupboards, etc. Never leave a chip pan or frying pan on the cooker unattended – oil will self-ignite when over-heated.

Electricity. **Never take electrical appliances – heater, radio, etc. – into the bathroom. Check that you have the correct wiring and fuses for your appliances.** Switch off or remove plugs of appliances when not in use. As regards electric lights, make sure the bulb is the right wattage for the lampshade you are using and never plug appliances into a light socket. Never remove plugs from sockets by pulling on the wire – you will eventually pull the wire loose. Do not use adaptors – have extra points installed instead. Have electric wiring checked regularly. Remember that if your house was wired more than twenty-five years ago then the number of electrical appliances available then was much smaller than it is today and the load would have been comparatively light.

Gas. In case of failure of supply, turn off all pilot lights or the main cock. When the supply returns re-light all pilots, not forgetting the water heater in the bathroom. Have all gas appliances serviced annually.

Inflammable materials. Inflammable liquids should be stored away from the house, if possible; adhesive solvents should be stored in closed containers in a cool place. Don't use adhesives near a naked flame, even a gas pilot light; don't operate light switches when using adhesives.

- Use only non-flammable cleaning fluids.
- Keep matches away from children.
- Always have a plentiful supply of ashtrays – guests may smoke even if you don't.
- Never smoke in bed.
- Never make improvised repairs.

In general, always follow manufacturers' instructions for safe use. When buying new equipment bear fire risks in mind. Choose equipment designed to British Standards Institute specifications and with the seal of approval of the British Electrical Approvals Board. Check on the after-sales service. Remember that it could be risky to buy secondhand electric or oil appliances.

Pyjamas are much safer than flowing nightdresses. Children's nightdresses are required by law to be made of flame-retardant material. Don't use paper for making fancy-dress costumes.

When buying upholstered furniture check that the materials used are flame retardant.

It is a good idea to have a fire extinguisher in the home. Make yourself familiar with the instructions for its use, and have it checked regularly according to the manufacturer's directions.

Rather than having your own fireworks, go to an organized fireworks display. And if you do use fireworks, make sure that everyone knows and uses the fireworks code.

When away from home, in the office or on holiday, read the fire instructions and make sure that you know the escape routes in case of fire. Check that you know what the fire-alarm signal is and where the alarm and the fire extinguishers are.

Fire safety at night
- Tidy up before retiring.
- Place guards over open fires.
- Switch off heaters.
- Switch off appliances not in use and remove plugs from sockets.
- See that all cigarettes are out.
- Close doors.

What to do in case of fire

Have a plan of action prepared so that every member of the family knows what to do.

- Bring everyone in the house to the ground floor where they can leave safely.
- See the fire brigade is called at once. Don't assume that someone else has already done so.
- See that everybody is safe and that the fire brigade has been called *before* investigating the fire.
- Eliminate draughts which may fan the fire; close all doors and windows even in rooms away from the fire.

If cut off by fire

- Close the door of the room and any fanlight or other opening and block up any cracks with bedding, etc.
- Go to the window and try to attract attention.
- If the room fills with smoke, lean out of the window unless prevented by smoke and flame coming from a room below or near by. If you cannot lean out of the window, lie close to the floor where the air is clearer, until you hear the fire brigade.
- If you have to escape before the fire brigade arrives, make a rope by knotting together sheets or similar materials and tie it to a bed or other heavy piece of furniture.
- If you cannot make a rope and the situation becomes intolerable, drop cushions or bedding from the window to break your fall, get through the window feet first, lower yourself to the full extent of your arms and drop.
- If possible, drop from a position above soft earth. If above the first floor drop *only* as a last resort.

If clothing catches fire

A person whose clothes are on fire should be laid on the floor and rolled in blankets, rugs or a thick coat. If your own clothing catches fire, roll on the floor to extinguish the flames.

Dealing with small fires

Chip pan fires. Turn off the heat and cover with a lid or damp tea towel; do not pour water over the pan.

Electrical fires. Switch off the power either at the appliance or at the fusebox; water may then be used to extinguish the fire. Unplug the affected appliance before switching the power back on.

Smoke and toxic fumes

Smoke and toxic fumes from fires kill more people than fire itself. Many people have died from inhaling toxic fumes when the actual fire was of very small proportions.

Smoke will travel upwards until it meets the ceiling, when it will travel horizontally. If doors are left open it will pass through the openings and fill the rooms beyond, and in a relatively short time a whole building can be completely filled with smoke, even from quite a small fire.

Smoke from fire contains carbon monoxide, which is highly poisonous. Even more dangerous nowadays are the fumes from materials such as PVC, polyurethane foam, polystyrene and other modern materials. (See Chapter 6 on inhaled poisons.)

Anyone overcome by smoke must be removed immediately to a smoke-free area and artificial respiration applied, including cardiac compression if the heart has stopped. This should be maintained until the patient is breathing unaided or until medical help arrives. Get the victim to hospital as soon as possible.

Beware of entering a smoke-filled room and *keep as low as possible*, holding your breath. Remember that smoke rises.

Burns

The different degrees of burns are categorized as follows.

First degree burns: identified on the skin by redness, mild swelling and some stinging pain. They can be caused by too much sun, brief contact with hot objects, hot water or steam. They injure only the outer layer of skin.

Second degree burns: these are deeper, penetrating to the second layer of skin. They may appear red or mottled, and the skin often is blistered. Swelling may last for several days and the surface of the skin may be wet because of escaping plasma. These burns can be caused by deep sunburn, hot liquids, flash burns from burning liquid and other sources of high heat.

Third degree burns: these go even deeper, destroying the skin all the way down to the third layer of fatty tissue below the two tough outer layers. The burn may look white or charred. Longer contact with very hot substances results in the most serious kinds of burns, which actually destroy the skin. Third degree burns may be less painful than second degree because the nerve endings in the skin are often destroyed.

Depending on the seriousness and extent of the burns, the care of a doctor may be required. In general, an adult who has second degree burns over 15 per cent of his body (10 per cent in a child) or more should probably be hospitalized. If the burn is only mild sunburn, of course, this is not necessary. But if the burns are more severe, deep enough to blister the skin, a doctor should be called. Burns of the hands, feet and face also require prompt medical attention, except for minor finger or toe blisters. Facial burns may lead to swelling in the respiratory tract, which could cause breathing problems. This, of course, is a dangerous possibility and should be attended by a doctor immediately.

Treatment

You can help a burn victim, even though there isn't much you can do to give him complete treatment for serious burns. It's your job to try to relieve pain, see that you avoid further danger as best you can, prevent contamination and infection, treat for shock, soothe the patient and call for medical help.

First degree burns usually require little treatment. You can relieve pain by applying cold water to the burned area, or by submerging it in cold water. Another method is to put on a shirt soaked in cool water, which will cool the burn as the water evaporates. A soothing ointment helps relieve minor burns. A dry dressing may be applied to prevent further exposure or to protect skin from abrasive clothing.

Second degree burns should be treated with cold water (not iced) until the pain is relieved. Fast cooling can reduce damage from the heat in the lower layers of skin. Gently blot the skin dry with a clean towel and cover it with a clean, dry dressing. Do not try to break blisters or remove pieces of skin. Do *not* use an antiseptic preparation, ointment, spray or home remedy on a severe burn. Leave it dry until medical care is obtained.

If an arm or leg has been burned, it should be kept elevated. Your patient should not be allowed to put pressure on burned areas of his back, elbows, legs or heels for long periods of time. If the legs or feet have been burned, bed rest is essential, even if the areas are small. Healing can be delayed dangerously in all wounds of the legs and feet if they are abused.

Once again, second degree burns that cover large areas (15 per cent in adults, 10 per cent in children) should have hospital care. Any second degree burn of the hand, foot or face also requires medical care.

Third degree burns are much more serious, of course, and should also be given prompt professional medical attention.

Don't remove charred clothing that is stuck to the burn. Instead, cover the burned areas with a clean dressing, or a clean sheet or other household linen. If your patient's hands are burned, keep them higher than his heart. Burned feet and legs should be kept elevated and the victim shouldn't be allowed to walk.

Victims with burns on the face should sit up or be propped up, and you must keep careful watch for breathing difficulty. Keep your patient's airway open.

It is essential to get the patient to hospital as fast as possible; if medical help is more than an hour away and your patient is conscious and not vomiting, you may give him a weak solution of salt and soda (one level teaspoonful of salt and half a level teaspoonful of baking soda in a quart of cool water). Do not give him alcohol. Have him sip it slowly, about half a glass over fifteen minutes – only half as much for a child and half as much again for an infant. If he vomits, don't give him more to drink.

Aspirin or similar home medication may be given for pain, and remember to reassure your patient. Burn victims are naturally very upset and need your tenderness.

Do not put iced water on burns; the cold can intensify a shock reaction. A cold pack may be applied to burned hands, face or feet, but don't make it icy cold. Don't put salt in the water and do not immerse burned parts in iced water.

Never apply ointment, burn preparations, grease or other home remedies to serious burns. They may cause complications, and they'll interfere with later treatment by a doctor.

If the victim has been rescued from a burning building he may also need treatment for *carbon monoxide poisoning* (see page 78).

Chemical burns need first aid fast. You must quickly flush away the chemical with lots of water. Use a shower or garden hose if you can. Immediate washing is better than any other treatment and should go on for at least five minutes. Get rid of clothing over the burned places.

If there are instructions for burns caused by the chemical printed on the label, follow them. You may use rubbing alcohol as a final rinse on carbolic acid burns on the skin. On alkali burns continue to wash with plain water until the soapy, 'slippery' feel is gone from the skin.

Burns of the eye. Acid burns on the eye should be flushed with lots of water on the face, eyelid and eye for fifteen minutes. If only one eye has been burned, make sure the washing water doesn't get into the unaffected eye. Pour the water from the inside corner of the burned eye outward, holding the lid open. Never use any chemical neutralizing agent in the eye – the resulting chemical interaction may produce a further burn as heat is released.

Get medical attention at once.

Cover the eye with a clean dressing, but don't use cotton wool; the fibres may get into the eye. Don't let your patient rub his eye; it can cause further injury. Give your patient aspirin if he complains of pain.

Alkali burns of the eye (laundry and dishwashing detergent and other cleaning solutions) are becoming frequent as these products come into widespread use. Again, don't let your patient rub the solution into his eye. Flush the face with lots of water, holding the lid open and washing the eye for at least thirty minutes. If there are particles of dry chemicals floating on the eye, lift them off carefully and gently with sterile gauze, a clean handkerchief or dry facial tissue. Use no chemical neutralizing agents – only clear water. Seek prompt medical attention.

Burns

What to look for

Carbon monoxide poisoning from inhaled smoke
Skin turns cherry red.

First degree burns
Skin redness, mild swelling and some stinging pain. Only outer layer of skin is damaged.

Second degree burns
Deeper. Penetration to second layer of skin. Swelling, blisters and moisture of escaping plasma

Third degree burns
Penetration down to third layer of skin and deeper. Burned areas look white or charred.

What to do

Treat before burns. Get victim into fresh air. If not breathing give mouth-to-mouth respiration.

Relieve pain by applying cold water. A soothing ointment may be applied. A dry dressing to prevent chafing if necessary.

Treat with cold water (not iced) until pain relieved. Cover with dry dressing. *Do not use salves or ointments. Leave burn dry.* If an arm or leg has been burned, it should be kept elevated.

Do not try to remove charred clothing that adheres to burn. Make sure patient's airway is open. If help is long way off and patient is conscious and not vomiting, give weak solution of salt and baking soda – one teaspoonful salt and half a teaspoonful soda to a quart of water – to be sipped slowly. Stop if he starts to vomit. Aspirin or similar remedy may be given for pain. *No salve or grease on burn.*

Chemical burns

Flush away chemical with lots of water. Get rid of clothing over burned areas. Use hose, shower, bucket.

Acid burns of the eye

Flush with lots of water on face, eyelid and eye for 15 minutes. Pour water from inside corner of eye outward, holding eyelid open. Do not let patient rub eyes. Get to doctor as soon as possible.

Alkali burns of the eye

Flush with water on eye, lid and face for 30 minutes. Get medical attention.

Action sequence for burns

If smoke has been inhaled get victim into fresh air. Give mouth-to-mouth respiration if necessary.

Treat all burns with flushings of cold (not iced) water.

Do not put ointment or salve on second and third degree burns. Doctor will make this decision.

Do not try to pull charred clothing from burns.

Keep burned arms and legs elevated higher than heart.

Make sure airway remains open. Keep watch for shock.

Aspirin or similar remedy may be given for pain for all burns.

A weak solution of salt and baking soda in water may be given to serious burn victims if hospital care will be delayed for an hour or more. Stop if patient begins to vomit.

Burn victims are naturally **very upset**. Give comfort and aid and reassure that help is on way. Watch for shock symptoms.

10. Childbirth

After all the pain and suffering we've described, it's time to look at one of life's miracles – the birth of a baby.

Birth is, of course, a natural and normal function for women, and usually occurs in hospital, or at home under the supervision of a midwife or doctor. Occasionally, however, the woman is in the wrong place at the wrong time. She isn't ready when the baby is.

Even so, most births follow their natural course, with mother and baby doing very well. Nevertheless, sudden births call for a quick response from people who are willing and capable of helping. This is a delicate time, and if you appear competent and confident both the mother and you will remember the event with warmth. Of course, the mother is embarrassed. She has been caught off guard. Try to arrange as much privacy as possible. Be gentle and reassuring. Get her trust. It will make things much easier for you both.

The first thing you'll need to decide when you come on a woman who apparently is about to give birth is how much time there is. Do you have time to take her to the hospital or should you prepare to deliver the child on the spot?

1. Ask the mother if she is having her first baby. Ask her how long she has been in labour. Ask her if she feels she has to strain or move her bowels. If she is having her first baby and she has not been in labour long, there probably is enough time to get her to a hospital. The average length of labour for a first baby is fifteen hours but it is considerably shorter for subsequent babies. But if the woman feels that she must strain or move her bowels this means that the baby has moved from the uterus into the birth canal, a reliable sign that birth is imminent.

2. You should examine the vaginal opening for crowning, the start of the appearance of the baby's head. If the exposed area of the baby's head is smaller than a fifty-pence piece and the mother is having her first baby, you'll probably have time to get her to the hospital. If the mother has already had children and the crowning is four inches wide or more, stand by, because delivery will probably occur in a few minutes.

If the labour contractions are about two minutes apart and the mother is straining or pushing down with contractions, crying out constantly and perhaps warning that the baby is coming, she's almost certainly right. You should be ready to assist in a delivery.

Never try to hold back the delivery of a baby by pushing on its head or telling the mother to cross her legs. The consequences can be fatal. Never put your fingers into the birth canal. Allow the delivery to proceed without interference until the baby's head has emerged fully.

Arrange for all the privacy you can and have the mother lie on her back, knees bent, feet flat and thighs separated widely. She can lie on the floor, on the seat of a car, on the ground, on any flat surface. Place clean cloths, clothing or newspapers under her buttocks. Wash your hands, if you can. If you can find a helper, have him stand by the woman's head to help and comfort her. Have a pan or pail ready, if you can, and have your helper guard against airway obstruction in case there is vomit.

If somebody can get a doctor on the phone so he can relay instructions to you, wonderful. Now get ready!

As the infant's head emerges, be ready to guide and support it with your hands to keep it from becoming contaminated with blood, mucus and other material. If the bag of waters breaks now, birth will take place fast, and, remember, a baby is slippery. If the baby's head appears with bag unbroken, tear it with your fingers to let the fluid escape.

(If the bag of waters breaks and the umbilical cord protrudes into the birth canal, this is dangerous. It doesn't happen often, but if it does the mother must be taken to a hospital immediately. She should remain in a jack-knife knee-to-chest position to relieve pressure on the cord so that the infant's blood supply won't be shut off.)

Usually the head will emerge face down. Check it to make sure the umbilical cord – which looks like a thick soft white rope about twenty inches long – isn't wrapped around the infant's neck. If it is, gently but quickly slip it over the baby's head. If the cord is wrapped around the baby's neck too tightly to remove, you must cut it immediately, at least four inches away from the baby's body, to prevent strangulation. Squeeze the cut ends with gauze, cloth or your fingers until they can be tied. (See below for how to tie and cut.)

Keep supporting the head as the baby is delivered. As the shoulders pass through the birth canal, the baby turns so that it is facing the mother's thigh. This turning makes the passage of the shoulders through the opening easier. The upper shoulder usually delivers first, sometimes with difficulty. To help, gently guide the baby's head downwards. Do not use force. Then guide the head upwards and this will help the emergence of the other shoulder.

Remember, a baby is very slippery, soft and delicate at birth. Even its head is soft, so always handle with great care.

Now the baby should emerge fast.

Your next task is to help the infant start breathing. Keep it warm and, although it may be blue, within a minute or two it should start breathing, crying and gradually turning a rosy pink.

To help, lower the baby's head and raise the feet, grasping the ankles with your hand. Wipe out the mouth and nose just enough to make certain there are no obstructions. If the infant is not crying, rub its back or flick your thumb and forefinger against the bottom of its feet. If it still isn't breathing, give artificial respiration through its mouth and nose with gentle puffs every three seconds.

When it is breathing well, wrap the baby and lay it down with its head extended back and a pad under its shoulders to keep the airway open. The mother may want to hold the baby on her stomach and this is fine, but watch the cord. It should be kept slack.

It is quite all right to leave the infant attached to the afterbirth by the umbilical cord. It's better to do this than to cut the cord with unclean instruments or to tie the cord improperly, but if cutting the cord is desirable, wait, if you can, until all pulsations in the cord have stopped, which should take about five minutes. Use a new razor blade or boiled scissors. Boil new white shoelaces, if you have them, or narrow strips of cloth to get them clean.

The cord must be tied four to six inches from the body of the baby, so that nothing can pass through it. A second tie should be about eight inches from the baby. The cord must not be cut closer than four inches from the baby's body. Use a new razor blade or boiled scissors to cut the cord *between the ties*. In a few days the cord end will dry up and fall off at the baby's navel.

About twenty minutes after the delivery of the baby the mother will discharge the placenta, or afterbirth, which is a messy affair. If the birth seems normal, without complications, delay the trip to the hospital so that the mother can discharge the placenta without the discomfort and mess of doing so in a moving vehicle.

Be patient when waiting for the delivery of the afterbirth; don't pull on the cord or push hard on the mother's stomach to hurry things along. As the afterbirth emerges, place your hand on the mother's lower abdomen and massage the uterus gently but firmly for a few minutes. This will help cause the uterus to contract and control bleeding. Keep this up every five minutes for at least an hour or until the mother is seen by a doctor.

When the placenta is expelled, wrap it in a towel or a bag so that it can be taken to the hospital with the mother. Doctors will want to examine it to make sure that all of it has been delivered from the mother's body.

After delivery of the baby, clean the mother's vaginal opening with a clean moist towel or soapy water poured from above, towards the rectum. Lay a sanitary towel or a clean cloth over the vagina. Give the mother tea, coffee or something else to drink and keep her warm and as comfortable as possible.

Some bleeding (about half a pint) is normal during the delivery, but if it continues later you should change the loose pads over the vagina and encourage the mother to keep her legs together to help slow the flow.

Do *not* attempt to clean off the white, greasy protective coating covering the baby's skin. Do *not* wash its eyes, ears or nose. The newborn baby is wet and small and loses body heat dangerously quickly. Wrap him in a blanket immediately and place him next to the mother for warmth.

Keep mother and child comfortable by replacing soiled linen and performing what acts of kindness you can. Wipe the mother's face with a clean cloth and perhaps rubbing alcohol. Let her know that she and her child are special – they've both just been through a great deal.

If there are complications at the birth, you must try to get the mother to the hospital at once. Sometimes the baby does not present its head first, but perhaps its buttocks (this is called a breech birth), or an arm or a leg. There's not much you can do to help except to encourage the mother and hope that the delivery takes place without harm to mother or child. If it is a multiple birth, your task is the same, taking care of both infants – and working twice as hard!

If you have time to gather supplies for a birth that is imminent, here is what you should have on hand: newspapers, plastic bags, clean towels, one or two sheets, a set of sterile cord ties, a new razor blade in its protective wrapper (single edge is best), alcohol, scissors, sanitary towels, a receiving blanket for the baby, a nappy and safety pins. If the mother-to-be is going for a long car ride, have her wear a nightgown or slip and a warm dressing-gown. Place a sanitary towel or a folded cloth between her thighs to absorb secretions. Take a torch.

Childbirth

What to look for

Birth appears imminent. Mother feels strain, need to move bowels. Baby has moved into birth canal. Labour contractions now only 2 minutes apart.

Crowning. Exposed area of baby's head appears in vaginal opening. If larger than 50-pence piece, baby ready to start. Let delivery proceed as head emerges.

If bag of waters breaks now, the delivery will go fast.

If head appears and bag is unbroken

As shoulders emerge, baby turns to face mother's thigh – upper shoulder emerges first, then lower shoulder.

Remainder of baby will move fast.

Baby should start breathing and crying. Face will be bluish at first, then turn rosy with crying. Help the baby to breathe.

What to do

Wash hands. Have supplies ready. Prepare mother for delivery. Flat on back, knees raised, feet flat and thighs separated. Place clean cloths or newspapers under mother's buttocks.

Do not interfere with natural developments. Stand by to help in delivery. Have someone by side of mother's head if possible to calm her and check her airway.

Baby will be slippery; be ready to handle surely and gently.

Tear bag open with fingers to release fluid.

Gently guide baby's head down to assist shoulder exit. Then move head up to help other shoulder out.

Be prepared to hold it – slippery.

To help it breathe, lower head and grasp ankles. Wipe out mouth and nose, rub its back or flick thumb and forefinger against bottom of feet. If still not breathing, give artificial respiration by gently blowing

	puffs of air into mouth and nose every 3 seconds.
Baby is crying and breathing well.	Wrap in cloth and lay with head extended back to breathe easily. Watch that umbilical cord is not tight or stretched. Keep slack. Keep baby warm – prevent loss of heat.
After delivery, mother will discharge placenta (afterbirth) after about 20 minutes.	When placenta is expelled, wrap in towel for hospital examination.
Umbilical cord may remain attached to infant if it is going to hospital.	Cord will be cut in hospital under more sterile conditions.
If head emerges with umbilical cord wrapped once about baby's neck.	Gently unwrap cord from around baby's neck.
If cord is wrapped tightly around baby's neck.	Cord must be cut immediately, lest baby strangle. Cut with pair of scissors that have been boiled to sterilize, or new razor blade. Tie cord 4 inches from baby as quickly as possible.
To cut cord after baby has been delivered under normal circumstances	Wait until pulsations stop (after 5 minutes). Use strips of cloth that have been boiled. Tie one strip around cord, about 4 inches from baby's body, tightly. The second strip about 8 inches from baby's body, tightly. Cut through umbilical cord between ties (no closer than 4 inches from baby's body).

As afterbirth emerges from the mother

Place hand on mother's lower stomach and gently massage. This will cause uterus to contract and will help control bleeding. Continue this every 5 minutes for one hour until doctor arrives.

After delivery of the baby

Clean mother's vaginal opening with clean, moist towel or soapy water poured from above towards rectum. Lay a sanitary towel or other clean cloth over the vagina.

Some bleeding is normal (about half a pint) during delivery, but if it continues later, change loose pads over vagina and encourage mother to keep legs together to help slow the flow of blood.

Do not attempt to clean off white, greasy protective covering on the baby's skin. *Do not* wash his eyes, ears or nose. Keep him warm by covering and placing close to mother.

Keep mother and baby comfortable by replacing soiled linen and being kind.

Wipe mother's face with clean cloth or some rubbing alcohol. Give her tea or coffee if she likes.

11. Sudden Illness and Other Emergencies

Stroke

A stroke can happen to any of us at any time, although they are more likely to occur in older people. A stroke usually means a rupture of a blood vessel in the brain or formation of a clot in the brain that retards circulation of the blood. We already know that the brain needs a great deal of blood to function normally.

Signs of a stroke may include unconsciousness and other, more specific signs, such as paralysis or weakness in one side of the body, including the facial muscles, difficulty in breathing and swallowing, loss of bladder and bowel control, unequal size of the pupils and inability to talk or slurred speech.

In a minor stroke the victim usually remains conscious and other symptoms are less pronounced.

Of course you should seek medical help immediately, and hospitalization will usually be necessary. Meanwhile, you should see that your patient's airway is kept open, place him on his side so that secretions will drain from his mouth, give him fluids if he is fully conscious and able to swallow, but discontinue if he vomits or becomes unconscious.

Convulsions

A convulsion or fit is a fearsome thing to see, unless you are familiar with what it means and how you can help. The victim usually experiences rigid muscles, jerking movements, bluish discoloration of his face, perhaps a foaming at the mouth, drooling and then gradual relaxation, after which he becomes sleepy and disoriented for a while.

During the fit, the victim will stop breathing, he may bite his tongue and lose bladder and bowel control.

Before a convulsion the victim may get a brief warning sensation and others may see a sudden paleness on his face or confused behaviour.

Mouth-to-nose respiration is not possible because of muscle rigidity, and the mouth is rigidly closed because of contraction.

Try to keep the victim from hurting himself during the seizure by loosely restraining the patient's arms and legs and supporting him on his side, allowing secretions to drain from the mouth. Inserting a twisted cloth between the patient's teeth may prevent him biting his tongue and choking on it too. Keep the airway open, so that when the fit passes the victim may breathe without obstruction. Then allow him to sleep or rest. Effective treatment has been developed by medical science; make sure that your patient sees a doctor.

Electrical emergencies

As with many of the other emergencies dealt with in this book, taking sensible precautions will prevent many accidents from happening in the first place. Even domestic mains voltage can kill, so treat it with respect. Don't use worn flexes. Don't leave trailing flexes or run them under a rug or carpet. Never take electrical appliances into the bathroom or touch a switch with wet hands. Always switch off appliances before tampering with them or unplugging them. Don't pull on the flex to remove a plug from a socket.

An electric shock is dangerous; it can paralyse the body's breathing centre in the brain and can cause unconsciousness or even death. Whether the shock is caused by wiring in the home, high tension wires outside, lightning or anything else the victim will need your help.

But be careful. If the victim is in contact with an electric current **do not approach him or touch him until you're certain that the current has been switched off**. Remember that damp ground will conduct electricity.

If it is not possible to switch off the current it may be possible to hook or push a live wire out of the way with a long wooden or plastic (*not metal*) stick. If out of doors, stand on your coat – if dry – or anything else which is a good insulator. (Rubber boots are the best protection of all.)

Try to keep the victim still until medical help arrives. If he isn't breathing, artificial respiration may be necessary. Leave the treatment of electric burns to medical personnel.

If electricity wires should fall across a car, the occupants should stay inside until trained help arrives. If fire or some other emergency forces the occupants to leave the 'wired' car, they must get clear without touching the ground or anything else outside the car while they are still in contact with the car. It is also vital to avoid 'grounding' the car. A safe method is for the person in the front seat to open the passenger door as wide as possible, being careful that it does not touch the ground or anything else which will conduct electricity. The passengers should then leave – one at a time – through this one door, in the following manner. Keep both feet inside the car and slide to the edge of the seat, fold your arms, move your head out from under the roof and then jump clear of the car with one intensive effort.

Diabetic shock

There are two kinds of crises relating to diabetes.

Hyperglycaemia means that there is too much sugar in the blood. There isn't much you can do for a victim of this kind of illness except to be able to recognize its onset and get the victim to medical care fast.

The victim may be drowsy for some time before the shock sets in. His breathing may become deep and rapid and his breath may have a peculiar fruity odour. He may become unconscious. You should look for a card in his wallet or an identification tag identifying him as a diabetic.

Immediate hospital treatment is necessary.

Hypoglycaemia means too little sugar in the blood. It may be caused by an overdose of insulin, a failure to eat after taking insulin, unusual exercise, hunger or emotional stress.

The victim may faint when his blood sugar falls. He may first be hungry with a gnawing sensation in his stomach. He may experience weakness, dizziness, cold sweating, paleness, tremors or dim eyesight, or he may display unusual behaviour. He may appear 'drunk'.

You must raise your patient's blood sugar as fast as you can. Sweets, sugar, soft drinks, fruit juice or anything else sweet is usually effective and may prevent unconsciousness. If your patient is unconscious, you can't feed him. You must get him to a hospital fast.

Heat

Excessive heat can upset the body in a number of ways ranging from mild discomfort to serious illness and even death.

Heat stroke is due to failure of the heat controlling mechanism and may occur as a result of exposure to heat or may complicate a feverish illness. The body temperature may reach 106°F, or even higher. The skin will get hot, red and dry because the sweating mechanism fails. The pulse will be rapid and strong and the victim may lose consciousness.

Your job is to cool your patient's body until 102°F is reached. Move him to a cool area immediately, then sponge his bare skin with cool water, or put him in a bath of cold water until his temperature goes down. Fans and air conditioners will help cool him. Don't give him stimulants. Prompt medical care is essential. This is a true emergency.

Heat cramps are muscular pains and spasms brought on by loss of salt in the body, usually by profuse sweating. The victim's legs and abdomen are likely to be affected first, and he could suffer from mental confusion and even convulsions.

Give him sips of salt water (one teaspoonful of salt per pint), half a glass every fifteen minutes over about an hour. Gently massage his muscles to help relieve spasms.

Heat exhaustion is caused by too little intake of water to make up for loss of fluid through sweating. The victim feels tired and weak, and he may collapse. The skin becomes pale and clammy, and the victim may complain of nausea, dizziness and cramps.

Give him salt water (formula above), have him lie down and raise his feet several inches, loosen his clothing, apply cool cloths, fan him. If he vomits, don't give him any more to drink.

Your patient should rest for several days.

Cold

Exposure to cold is especially dangerous in babies and the elderly, whose temperature regulating mechanisms are unreliable. General lowering of body temperature is termed hypothermia and local damage by cold to the tissues of exposed extremities is termed frostbite.

The elderly may be especially prone to hypothermia because of malnutrition, insufficient heating in the house and loss of mobility from arthritis or paralysis. But mountaineers exposed to bad weather conditions when fatigued and drunks lying overnight in a gutter, insensible to the cold and unable to move, may also be victims of hypothermia. It can occur even in the absence of cold if the metabolic rate is depressed by endocrine disorders.

Hypothermia. There is a loss of surface heat to the environment and then cooling of the deep tissues and organs. Rectal temperature drops to 80–90°F.

The patient becomes confused, drowsy and at around 86°F will become comatose. The pulse and respiratory rate are slow and blood pressure low. Ultimately death occurs. An ordinary household thermometer will not register the low temperatures of hypothermia.

Treat by warming the body with warm blankets and warm drinks until medical help is obtained. *Do not* give alcohol, rub the victim's skin or place a hot water bottle against him.

If you are going walking in the hills make sure that you take adequate food and clothing, even if the weather is fine when you set out. If one of your party shows symptoms of hypothermia, stop, send for help, and do what you can to keep the victim warm and his morale high.

Frostbite. Ears, nose, chin, fingers and toes are most often affected; the affected parts are numb and white and may or may not be painful; if not treated gangrene may set in.

Urgent medical treatment is needed but meantime ensure general protection from hypothermia as above and local thawing of the affected part by removal of any constrictive clothing or rings and warming with blankets. Do not rub or massage the frostbitten area.

Sudden Illness and Other Emergencies

What to look for

Stroke

Paralysis or weakness on one side of body. Difficulty in breathing and swallowing, loss of bladder and bowel control, eye pupils unequal size, slurred speech. Unconscious.

Convulsions

Patient may go very pale or have confused behaviour before seizure. Rigid muscles, jerky movements, bluish colour of face, foaming at mouth, drooling. Then gradual relaxation, sleepiness.

Electric shock

Can paralyse breathing centre in brain and cause unconsciousness.

Diabetic shock

Hyperglycaemia: too much sugar in the blood. Drowsy before shock sets in. Breathing deep and rapid. Breath has fruity odour.

What to do

Seek medical help immediately. Place victim on side to drain secretions. Make sure airway is open.

May bite tongue or stop breathing. Prevent biting by inserting twisted cloth between teeth. **Get medical help**. Keep patient on side and maintain airway so patient may breathe when seizure ends.

Don't touch if victim still connected to current. When disconnected, treat as in shock cases. If not breathing, give mouth-to-mouth respiration. Also cardiac compression. Leave electrical burns to professionals. **Get to hospital.**

Get medical help fast. Refer to Chapter 5. Check wallet for diabetic identity card.

Hypoglycaemia: not enough sugar in the blood. Very hungry, weak, dizzy, cold sweats, pale, tremors, fainting. Many act 'drunk'.

Must raise patient's blood sugar immediately with sweets, sugar, soft drinks, fruit juice or anything sweet to prevent unconsciousness. Get to hospital fast.

Heat stroke

Body temperature will climb to 106°F or more. Skin red and dry. No perspiration, pulse rapid, strong. Victim may lose consciousness.

Cool patient's body by sponging with cold water. Put into bath of cold water. Get medical help fast – this is life threatening. Don't give stimulants.

Heat cramps

Muscular pains and spasms, mental confusion, convulsions.

Give salt water (1 teaspoon per pint). Massage muscles.

Heat exhaustion

Victim feels tired and weak, may collapse. Skin pale and clammy. Nausea, dizziness, cramps.

Give salt water as above, but not if vomiting. Get him to lie down, raise feet, loosen clothing, apply cool cloths, fan.

Hypothermia

Patient confused, drowsy, then comatose. Pulse and breathing slow.

Warm patient's body with warm blankets and warm drinks. Get medical help.

Frostbite

Affected area will look white or grey – it will feel numb, but may not be painful.

Thaw frozen part with warm blankets. Do not rub the frostbitten area. Get medical help.

Action sequence for emergencies

Stroke
Place on side to drain secretions from mouth. Make sure airway is open. **Get medical help fast.**

Convulsions
Prevent patient from biting tongue, if possible with a twisted cloth between his teeth. Keep patient on his side. Keep airway open so patient may breathe when seizure ends. **Get medical help fast.**

Electric shock
Do not touch if the victim is still connected to the current. When disconnected, treat as shock case. If not breathing give mouth-to-mouth assisted breathing. Do cardiac compression if no pulse. Leave electrical burns to medical personnel.

Diabetic shock
If conscious, diabetic can probably tell you what to do. Giving sugar (two lumps is enough) or something sweet will usually help, and can do little harm. **If unconscious, get the patient to hospital immediately.**

Heat stroke
Cool patient by sponging his body with cold water. Put into a bath of cold water. No stimulants. **Get to hospital fast.**

Heat cramps	Give salt water (1 teaspoon per pint) to sip. Gently massage muscles.
Heat exhaustion	Give salt water as above, unless he vomits. Get victim to lie down, raise feet, loosen clothing, apply cool cloths, fan.
Hypothermia	Warm with warm blankets and warm drinks. **Get medical help**.
Frostbite	Warm patient rapidly. Maintain respiration.

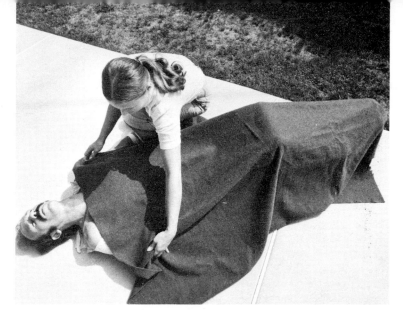

There isn't much you can do for the victim of a stroke. Keep your patient as warm and comfortable as you can. Keep calm, try to soothe him and send for professional help immediately.

Give a patient with heat stroke a good soaking with cool water, saturating his clothing. Don't be afraid to wet his hair, face and hands. This will help reduce his body temperature and cool his skin. It also helps to dampen towels or other material and place them on his body to hasten cooling.

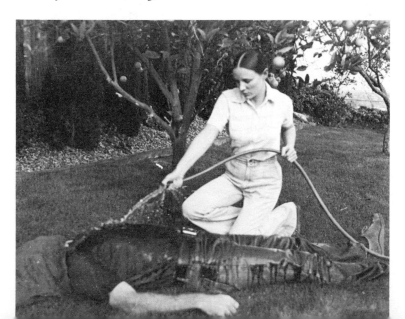

Appendix

First aid kit to carry in the car

Sterile adhesive plasters (Elastoplast, etc.)
Sterile 4 × 4 inch (10 × 10 cm) gauze pads
Small bar of soap
Antiseptic ointment
Plastic bottle of water for irrigation or washing
Small scissors
Tweezers for removing splinters
Roll of bandage, 1 inch (2.5 cm) wide
Triangular bandage for sling or bandage
Roll of stretch bandage
Torch
Single-edge razor blade
Two large safety pins

First aid kit for the home

Sterile adhesive plasters (Elastoplast, etc.)
Sterile 4 × 4 inch (10 × 10 cm) gauze pads
Small scissors
Antiseptic ointment
Roll of bandage, 1 inch (2.5 cm) wide
Tweezers for removing splinters
Syrup of ipecac, 1 oz (30 g) bottle
Triangular bandage for sling or bandage
Roll of stretch bandage
Telephone numbers of doctor, local hospital (casualty department) and nearest
  poison information service, close to the telephone

More about Penguins
and Pelicans

For further information about books available from Penguins please write to Dept EP, Penguin Books Ltd, Harmondsworth, Middlesex UB7 0DA.

In the U.S.A.: For a complete list of books available from Penguins in the United States write to Dept CS, Penguin Books, 625 Madison Avenue, New York, New York 10022.

In Canada: For a complete list of books available from Penguins in Canada write to Penguin Books Canada Ltd, 2801 John Street, Markham, Ontario L3R 1B4.

In Australia: For a complete list of books available from Penguins in Australia write to the Marketing Department, Penguin Books Australia Ltd, P.O. Box 257 Ringwood, Victoria 3134.

In New Zealand: For a complete list of books available from Penguins in New Zealand write to the Marketing Department, Penguin Books (N.Z.) Ltd, P.O. Box 4019, Auckland 10.

A Pelican Book

Alternative Medicines
A Guide to Natural Therapies

Andrew Stanway

Acupuncture . . . Alexander Technique . . . Biochemics . . . Herbal Medicine
. . . Homeopathy . . . Hypnosis . . . Macrobiotics . . . Osteopathy . . . Radionics
. . . Shiatsu . . . Sound Therapy . . . Yoga . . .

Alternative medicine is of growing interest and concern to millions of people
in the West who feel that conventional medicine cannot always supply
solutions to health problems.

This book is designed to offer information (often difficult to obtain from your
doctor) on thirty-two therapies. Written by a doctor who has taken care to
make his material as accessible as possible, it provides an excellent and
objective guide to the alternatives to conventional medicine.

A Penguin Reference Book

Medicines

A Guide for Everybody
Fourth Edition

Peter Parish

Incorporating new tables on oral contraception, a new chapter on drugs used to conquer cancer and a completely updated Pharmacopoeia.

Part One outlines the basic principles of drug use. Part Two analyses groups of drugs by their uses. Part Three has been extensively revised and up-dated for this edition and lists drugs alphabetically giving precautions, dosages and cross-references to Part Two.

Medicines of all kinds heal thousands and comfort millions, but few of us ever use them to maximum benefit. Yet much of the disappointment, the side-effects and the wasted money is avoidable if we understand enough either to cooperate with a doctor, or to medicate ourselves intelligently.

A Penguin Reference Book

The Penguin Medical Encyclopedia
Second Edition

Peter Wingate

'A highly commendable book which will no doubt go through many future editions' – *Journal of the Institute of Health Education*

Hippocrates asserted over two thousand years ago that a doctor must teach his patients to care for their own health. Until recently, however, most doctors have preferred to believe that patients can know too much.

This encyclopedia – which has been revised and brought up to date – is addressed to anyone who is concerned with the care of sick people and in particular to the patient himself, who should be the doctor's principal colleague. At the same time Dr Wingate (who regularly broadcasts on medical topics) is emphatic that it is not a 'Home Doctor' or do-it-yourself medical manual.

In hundreds of entries, running from *abdomen* to *zymosis*, he deals with the body and mind in health and sickness, with drugs and surgery, with the history, institutions and vocabulary of the profession and with many other aspects of medical science. In the course of these Dr Wingate clearly explains the principles involved in the diagnosis and treatment of a thousand and one illnesses, from the inconvenience of baldness to the rigours of cancer.

A Penguin Handbook

First Aid for Hill Walkers and Climbers

Jane Renouf and Stewart Hulse

Each year more and more people take to the hills, and each year the toll of deaths and injuries increases. Because it may take hours for help to arrive, the first-aider may, in some cases, hold the survival of the victim entirely in his hands.

This practical, sensible and long-needed manual will slip easily into a pocket or rucksack. It has been compiled with the aid of rescuers and experienced climbers and walkers from all over Britain. While not intended as a substitute for a first-aid course, it tells you how to deal with accidents on the mountainside and how to set about getting help in the most efficient and least panicky way: and, for easy reference the authors list the different accidents and illnesses in alphabetical order, ranging from asthma to vertigo.